D0907948

Points to Consider:
Responses to HIV/AIDS
in Africa, Asia and the Carribean

Paul,
Good to meet. Lots has been
accomplished. Still a
lot to do.

Published by
Adonis & Abbey Publishers Ltd
P.O. Box 43418
London
SE11 4XZ
http://www.adonis-abbey.com
Email: editor@adonis-abbey.com

First Edition, February 2008

Copyright 2007 © David Gisselquist

British Library Cataloguing-in-Publication Data
A catalogue record for this book is available from the British Library

ISBN: 9781905068265(HB)/9781905068456 (PB)

The moral right of the author has been asserted

All rights reserved. No part of this book may be reproduced, stored in a
retrieval system or transmitted at any time or by any means without the prior
permission of the publisher

Printed and bound in Great Britain

Points to Consider:
Responses to HIV/AIDS
in Africa, Asia and the Carribean

David Gisselquist

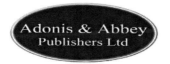

Table of Contents

List of Tables and Figures

Acknowledgements

This book is the product of eight years of research during which I have received more help and advice than anyone has any right to expect. Steve Minkin and Lucy Hancock encouraged me from 1999, when I began to look for information on blood exposures as risks for HIV infection. Yvan Hutin, Jules Millogo, Selma Khamassi, Lone Simonsen, Mark Miller, and many others whom I met through the Safe Injection Global Network, guided me with information and questions.

Much of the evidence and arguments in this book have been assembled in collaboration with research partners and co-authors of journal articles. For their many contributions to what is presented in these pages, I thank John Potterat, Mariette Correa, Francois Vachon, Garance Upham, Stuart Brody, Devon Brewer, Eric Friedman, Rich Rothenberg, Ernest Drucker, Valsa Madhava, Steven Q. Muth, Deodatta Gore, Lillian Salerno, Moses Okinyi, and Tobias Ounga.

The World Health Organization, South Africa's Human Sciences Research Council, Global Health through Education, Training and Service, Mariette Correa, Retractable Technologies, Inc., Hindustan Syringes and Medical Devices, Ltd., and Star Syringe, Ltd., provided occasional small grants for research and travel on topics related to this book.

The Hershey Medical Center and library staff, including Sharon Daugherty, Marie Fitzsimmons, and many others, provided access to journals and other research assistance.

John Gordon, Francois Vachon, Garance Upham, Mariette Correa, Brian Foley, Tom O'Connell, Jane Perry, Janine Jagger, David Sobel, Sarah Melendez, Robert Steinglass, Joe Lieberson and others not named read and criticized all or parts of early drafts, averting many errors. I'll claim the remaining errors.

I thank Vidyadhar Gadgil for preparing the manuscript for publication, and Jideofor Adibe at Adonis & Abbey for his support in bringing this book to market.

Finally, I thank my wife, Carol, for supporting my work on this topic for eight years, and for good advice on arguments and content.

David Gisselquist
December 2007

Glossary*

AIDS	acquired immunodeficiency syndrome
antibody	a molecule that bodies produce to target and control a specific virus, parasite, or toxin
BCG	Bacillus Calmette-Guerin, a vaccine against tuberculosis
CAR	Central African Republic
CDC	United States Centers for Disease Control and Prevention
CRF	circulating recombinant form
DPT	diphtheria, pertussis, tetanus
DRC	Democratic Republic of Congo
EPI	Expanded Programme on Immunization
HIV	human immunodeficiency virus
HIV-1	human immunodeficiency virus type 1
HIV-2	human immunodeficiency virus type 2
IDU	injection drug user
incidence	the rate at which an event, such as a new infection, occurs in a population; often given in events per 100 persons per year
MSM	men who have sex with men
POST	patient observed sterile treatment
prevalence	the proportion of a population that has a condition such as an infection at a specified time
sentinel survey	a survey to determine HIV prevalence in a population; surveys are characteristically anonymous (names are removed from samples before testing) and are repeated from year to year to see trends in prevalence
SIDA	syndrome d'immuno deficience acquise
SIGN	Safe Injection Global Network
SIV	simian immunodeficiency virus

UK	United Kingdom
UN	United Nations
UNAIDS	Joint United Nations Programme on AIDS
UNESCO	United Nations Educational, Scientific and Cultural Organization
UNICEF	United Nations Children's Fund
US	United States
USAID	United States Agency for International Development
virus	a large molecule that can reproduce inside living cells
WHO	World Health Organization

* For abbreviations which occur only once in the text, the full form is given immediately after the term in the text.

Chapter 1

IGNORING HIV FROM HEALTHCARE IN THE WORST AIDS EPIDEMICS

In countries with the worst HIV/AIDS epidemics, public messages about how to avoid HIV infection have given people incomplete information about risks. In most countries outside of sub-Saharan Africa, HIV infects far less than 1 percent of adults, and infections concentrate in injecting drug users (IDUs) and men who have sex with men (MSMs). However, in Africa, parts of the Caribbean, and a handful of countries in Asia and Oceania, HIV does not concentrate in IDUs and MSMs but rather invades the general population, creating what are called generalized epidemics.

In countries with generalized epidemics, HIV risk is a two-way street. Some people are infected by HIV from sexual exposures. Others are infected through blood exposures, including traces of HIV-contaminated blood on skin-piercing instruments reused without sterilization during medical injections, dental care, tattooing, and other healthcare and cosmetic procedures. The proportions of total 'traffic' coming from each direction are unknown.

Public health experts have known for decades that healthcare providers in much of Africa and Asia often reused syringes, needles, and other skin-piercing instruments without sterilization. In 1991, the World Health Organization (WHO) prepared a booklet advising United Nations (UN) employees 'living or traveling in areas where the level of medical care is uncertain' to

> ...take special precautions to avoid HIV transmission via blood...
> If you carry your own needles and syringes, make sure they are the ones used on you. If you are not carrying your own needles and syringes, avoid having injections unless they are absolutely necessary...
> Avoid tattooing and ear-piercing. Avoid any procedures that pierce the skin, such as acupuncture and dental work, unless they are genuinely necessary. Before submitting to any treatment that may give an entry point to HIV, ask whether the instruments to be used have been properly sterilized.[1]

In revisions of this booklet published in 1999 and 2004, UNAIDS provided similar warnings to UN employees and their families.[2]

In countries where WHO and UNAIDS warn UN staff to avoid HIV infection through blood exposures, neither WHO nor UNAIDS nor other international or national organizations have systematically extended similar warnings to the general public, thus providing incomplete information about risks. Not warning people about risks leads to avoidable HIV infections from overlooked blood exposures. Misinformation also contributes to stigma. HIV prevention messages that focus exclusively on sex and do not mention common blood exposures mislead people into believing that an HIV infection is a reliable sign of sexual misbehavior.

Women at risk

In countries where HIV infections concentrate in IDUs and MSMs, HIV infects several men for every woman. However, in generalized epidemics, especially in the worst ones, HIV infects more women than men (see Chapters 5 and 6). In Lesotho, for example, among adults aged 15–49 years, HIV infects 26 percent of women compared to 19 percent of men.

High HIV prevalence in women in generalized epidemics is hard to explain on the basis of their reported sexual behavior. Most HIV-positive women in Lesotho, as in other countries with generalized epidemics in Africa, Asia, or the Caribbean, report 0–1 sexual partners in the last year – sexual behavior that is conservative or average relative to other women in those countries, or in the US and Europe for that matter (see Chapter 7). Furthermore, among married women who are HIV-positive, more than half their husbands are HIV-negative in 9 of 17 countries with generalized epidemics (see Chapter 7).

Unexamined and uncontrolled risks

In the US, Europe, and many other countries, public awareness of risks of acquiring HIV infection from skin-piercing instruments led to public policies that reduced those risks to near zero. No country with reliable sterilization of medical instruments has a generalized epidemic. This poses the question: how much does HIV transmission through blood exposures in healthcare and cosmetic services contribute to generalized epidemics?

Unfortunately, no one knows. HIV is relatively easy to track – transmission requires sexual or blood-to-blood contact. It does not pass through casual contact (like measles), through the air (like tuberculosis), or through mosquitoes (like malaria). Yet 23 years after scientists developed tests for HIV infection in 1984, no one has traced HIV infections in generalized epidemics to see how many are coming from blood exposures. The lack of investigations makes it hard to stop HIV transmission through healthcare, because no one knows what procedures and which clinics are responsible.

In recent years, the AIDS epidemic has come into better focus. In most countries around the world, the number of new infections per year has fallen from peaks reached in the period 1985–2000. At the same time, treatment is getting better and is reaching more people in low- and middle-income countries. In more than thirty countries with generalized epidemics in Africa, Asia, and the Caribbean, national surveys during 2001–07 have improved—and lowered—estimates of the numbers of people living with HIV infections. But even these lower estimates describe ongoing disasters. In the absence of a vaccine— which is years away, at best—understanding how HIV infects so many people in generalized epidemics is crucial to controlling them.

Why have AIDS experts ignored HIV from unsafe healthcare?

Some of the earliest AIDS research in Africa in the mid-1980s found evidence for HIV transmission during healthcare, including many HIV-infected children with HIV-negative mothers (see Chapter 5). Despite this evidence, beginning from the late 1980s HIV prevention messages for the general public said little or nothing about infections from use of unsterile instruments during healthcare.

But the issue did not go away. During 1999-2003, after WHO had all but ignored HIV transmission through healthcare for more than a decade, people inside and outside WHO presented disturbing new estimates of the numbers of HIV infections from blood exposures during healthcare (Chapter 8). For example, a review of evidence commissioned by UNAIDS concluded in 2002 that 'contaminated [medical] injections may cause between 12% and 33% of new HIV infections' in Africa.[3] Also in 2002, a WHO team using other evidence estimated that medical injections caused 5 percent of new HIV infections in the world.[4]

What happened next? UNAIDS suppressed the high (12–33 percent) estimate by not releasing the report. But even with WHO's lower (5 percent) estimate, medical injections alone were infecting several hundred thousand people per year. To find and stop HIV transmission through healthcare, a crucial next step was to look for those estimated infections and for the clinics and procedures that were doing the damage. But that did not happen (see Chapter 9).

From this experience, and from the history presented in the following chapters, I think the major obstacle to recognizing and talking about HIV transmission through blood exposures in countries with generalized epidemics has been conflict of interest. For healthcare professionals, discussion and disclosure of HIV transmission through healthcare could bring public criticism, loss of public trust, loss of prestige, investigations, suits, and criminal charges. Many healthcare professionals have allowed such personal concerns to influence what they say. Conflict of interest has been especially influential and dangerous in many ex-colonies—and in foreign-funded health aid programs in ex-colonies—due to historic and continuing patterns of paternalism and elitism in public health management.

Healthcare professionals' lack of attention to HIV transmission through unsafe practices can be compared to the tobacco industry's attempt to mislead people about risks from smoking. For decades, the tobacco industry published shoddy research showing that smoking was safe. Fortunately, medical researchers—who did not have a conflict of interest with respect to cigarettes—did some honest research, and showed that smoking led to lung cancer and other health damage.

While medical researchers exposed dangers covered up by the tobacco industry, who will expose HIV transmission during healthcare? This is, of course, not an exact parallel – most healthcare professionals work for the common good, and many are saints. But some are not aware, and some people with good intentions can be distracted and misled by self-interest. Moreover, the epidemic's intersections with racial and sexual issues can confuse people – through unrecognized but nevertheless influential racial stereotypes, and through emotional reactions to relevant sexual and gender situations.

4

The purpose of this book

The purpose of this book is to challenge misinformation about risks in countries with generalized HIV epidemics, and to motivate the public, reporters, politicians, and lawyers in those countries to do what is necessary to protect themselves and to stop HIV transmission through blood exposures. To do so, this book presents a history of the HIV epidemic, with attention to blood exposures and to what public health managers have and have not done to protect people from HIV transmission through blood exposures.

The structure of the book

Chapter 2 begins with the passage of HIV from chimpanzees, gorillas, and sooty mangabeys to humans, and ends in 1960, when most countries in Africa achieved independence. Colonial healthcare programs spread bloodborne pathogens. Some of this was 'innocent,' because doctors were not aware of the risks.

Chapter 3 covers the silent expansion of HIV both in and outside Africa in the period 1960–81. During this period, public health managers in Africa recognized death and disease from bloodborne viruses (including the hepatitis B virus, which leads to liver disease, and the Ebola virus, which causes deadly hemorrhagic fever), but did not adequately address risks of transmitting these and other pathogens through reuse of medical instruments without sterilization.

Chapters 4 and 5 describe emerging ideas about AIDS from 1981, when doctors in California first recognized AIDS, to 1988, when the world's AIDS experts reached a consensus to overlook HIV transmission through healthcare in generalized epidemics. Chapter 4 deals with the period 1981–84, before the introduction of blood tests for HIV infection. Chapter 5 deals with the period 1984–88, when blood tests allowed people to see who and how many were infected, and to examine risks for HIV infection.

Chapters 6–9 cover the period from 1989 to 2007. During this period, the worst HIV epidemics developed in relatively wealthy and educated populations in Africa, while low-level generalized epidemics emerged in a handful of countries outside Africa (see Chapter 6). Chapter 7 examines weaknesses in the dialogue between AIDS experts and people in countries with generalized epidemics. Experts have not trusted and worked with HIV-positive adults to trace the sources of their infections and thereby to identify the risks that drive generalized epidemics. Chapter 8 reviews estimates of the proportion of HIV transmission through healthcare in generalized epidemics. (If you wish, you can skip some of the more technical parts of this chapter without losing the train of the argument in the rest of the book.) Chapter 9 describes long-term failure on the part of public health managers to address risks of HIV transmission through blood exposures in generalized epidemics.

Looking to the future, Chapter 10 considers how the public, aware of risks, could demand safe care. Money and budgets are secondary issues. Safe care does not have to be much more expensive, and in many situations it may even be cheaper – for example, patients can ask for pills instead of injections. Notably, safe healthcare does not wait for more foreign advice or money. By definition, the solution must be local, involving accountability to the local population.

Additional introductory comments

Several healthcare professionals who read early drafts of this book noted that colonial and post-colonial aid-financed healthcare programs in Africa and Asia reduced deaths and improved the quality of life. This is true: healthcare providers and programs *have* delivered substantial benefits. But do these benefits somehow balance or excuse the dis-benefits discussed in this book? Setting benefits side-by-side with dis-benefits proposes an implicit choice between unsafe healthcare and no healthcare. But there is a third choice: safe care. Medical schools teach doctors to 'first do no harm.' Medical ethics oblige doctors to warn patients about risks. There is no question that healthcare programs deliver benefits. The argument in this book is that healthcare should and could deliver fewer dis-benefits.

The book's topical focus on HIV transmission through healthcare guides the geographic focus on Africa, India, and other countries with generalized epidemics. This book sidesteps debates about HIV prevention among IDUs and MSMs, as well as the best policies and programs to prevent heterosexual transmission of HIV. The resolution of these debates one way or the other does not make healthcare safe, nor do initiatives for safe healthcare (as described in Chapter 10) threaten programs to stop HIV transmission through sex or IDU. Similarly, I endorse efforts to extend antiretroviral treatment to all people in low- and middle-income countries, but I leave to others debates about how best to do so.

This book refers to all HIV infections acquired from formal and informal healthcare as nosocomial infections (acquired or occurring in a hospital) or iatrogenic infections (from a doctor), even though some of the healthcare settings are markets or streets, and many healthcare providers who administer unsafe invasive procedures are not doctors, and some even have no medical qualifications.

---

[1] WHO. *AIDS and HIV infection: Information for United Nations employees and their families.* Geneva: WHO, 1991. Doc. no. WHO/GPA/DIR/91.9. p. 23.

[2] UNAIDS. *AIDS and HIV Infection: Information for United Nations employees and their families.* Geneva: UNAIDS, 1999; UNAIDS. *Living in a World with HIV and AIDS: Information for employees of the UN system and their families.* Geneva: WHO, 2004.

[3] Randerson J. 'WHO accused of huge HIV blunder', *New Scientist*, 2003, 180 (2424): 8–9.

[4] Hauri AM, Armstrong GL, Hutin YJF. 'The global burden of disease attributable to contaminated injections given in healthcare settings', *Int J STD AIDS*, 2004, 15: 7–16.

Chapter 2

THE AIDS EPIDEMIC BEGINS, 1920-60

Available evidence provides a pretty good picture of where and when the AIDS epidemic began. How and why it began when it did are questions for which there are so far no agreed answers but only competing hypotheses. These hypotheses deal not only with history, but are also linked to ideas about what currently drives HIV epidemics in Africa, Asia, and the Caribbean. Before discussing hypotheses for the origin of the HIV epidemic, it would be useful to review what is known about HIV's early history.

Clues to the early history of the AIDS epidemic

The AIDS epidemic began decades before doctors first recognized AIDS in 1981. In 1983, French scientists discovered HIV, the virus that causes AIDS. Tests based on HIV soon found similar viruses in African monkeys, and later in apes (chimpanzees and gorillas). These viruses have been named simian immunodeficiency viruses (SIVs). Monkeys and chimpanzees infected with SIVs in the wild seldom if ever get sick, which is common when a virus has lived with a host species for many years.

Tests based on HIV also discovered a closely related virus circulating in humans. This virus was named HIV type 2 (HIV-2), while the first HIV discovered was renamed HIV-1. HIV-2 transmits much less efficiently than HIV-1 (through blood, sex, and mother-to-child), has not spread much outside West Africa, and leads more slowly and less predictably to AIDS. Although HIV-2 has much less impact on human health than does HIV-1, the origin and early history of HIV-2 provide insights into the parallel origin and early history of HIV-1.

Much of what we know about the pre-1981 history of the AIDS epidemic comes from analyses of HIV and SIV molecules. Like other viruses, each HIV and SIV is a large molecule composed of a sequence of smaller molecules (nucleotides). For various reasons – including random errors during virus reproduction – these sequences change over time. Comparing one virus with others, those whose sequences are the most alike are the fewest years removed from a common 'parent' virus which lived and multiplied in a host years ago.

Moreover, estimates of the rate of change allow scientists to estimate the date of the most recent (last) common ancestor for any two HIVs and/or SIVs. From this information, they can draw viral 'family trees,' and can date the nodes which identify the last common ancestors of any two or more viruses.

HIV-1 origin and epidemic expansion to 1960

Where and when HIV-1 began

All HIV-1 molecules are more similar to – and thus more closely related to – SIV from chimpanzees and gorillas than to HIV-2 or to SIVs from other simian species. Hence, HIV-1 appears to have descended from SIV that passed from chimpanzees and gorillas to infect humans. (Once an SIV infects a human, it is an HIV. The change in name refers to the host. Whether SIV must change or evolve to transmit among humans is a matter of debate.)

All known HIV-1s can be sorted into three groups. The M (main) group accounts for well over 99 per cent of HIV-1 in the world. The O (outlier) group has been part of the HIV-1 epidemic in Cameroon and Gabon, but is rare in other countries. HIV-1 in the N (non-M, non-O) group has been found in a handful of people in Cameroon. Each of these three groups appears to have begun from a separate event in which SIV passed from a chimpanzee (twice) and a gorilla (once) to infect a human. The evidence for this is that HIV from each group is more similar to – and hence more closely related to – some of the SIV samples collected from chimpanzees and/or gorillas than to HIV from the other two groups.

All the SIV samples that are closest to HIV-1 in the M (main) and N groups have been collected from the chimpanzee sub-species, *Pan troglodytes troglodytes*, which ranges south of the Sanaga River in Cameroon, through Gabon and the Republic of Congo (hereafter identified as Congo) and east as far as the Congo river and its tributaries that define the northwest border of the Democratic Republic of Congo (DRC) (see the map of Africa in the Statistical Annex). More distantly related SIV has been found in the chimpanzee sub-species, *P.t. schweinfurthii*, which ranges east of the Congo River across DRC into Tanzania. Because chimpanzees are loath to cross rivers, these two sub-species, living on opposite sides of the Congo River, have bred

9

separately for an estimated 117,000 years.[1] SIV was circulating among chimpanzees before these two populations split, and has therefore been available to infect humans for well over 100,000 years.

In a remarkable bit of scientific sleuthing, scientists found close matches between SIV from the feces of wild chimpanzees living in southeast Cameroon and the HIV-1 M group.[2] Apparently, the virus that accounts for most of the world's HIV infections passed from a chimpanzee to a human somewhere in southeast Cameroon. The same study found other close matches between SIV from chimpanzees in south-central Cameroon and the HIV-1 N group.

In 2006, researchers reported SIV in gorilla feces collected in southern Cameroon.[3] From analyses of SIV sequences, the gorilla's SIV appears to be a branch of the viral tree for SIV from chimpanzees, which suggests that a gorilla many centuries ago somehow contracted SIV from a chimpanzee. Surprisingly, HIV-1 from the O group appears to be most closely related to SIV from gorillas. Apparently SIV from a gorilla passed to a human somewhere in or near southern Cameroon to begin the HIV-1 O group. So far none of the SIV sequences from gorillas are close enough to O group sequences to allow one to be more specific about where this might have occurred.

From differences between HIV-1 M group viruses, scientists have estimated the date of the most recent common ancestor of the M group. Five estimates range over the period from 1916 to 1937.[4] That is not the date when the SIV that begat the M group crossed to a human, but rather the date that an infected human – who may have been the first one infected, or someone later down the chain of infection – passed HIV to another to establish at least two lineages (chains of infection) that have survived and contribute to the current HIV-1 M group epidemic.

HIV-1 O group viruses are somewhat more diverse than M group viruses,[5] which suggests they have an older common ancestor. One estimated date for the most recent common ancestor of the O group is 1920.[6] The N group shows much less diversity than the M or O groups, and therefore appears to have descended from a more recent parent virus,[7] possibly in the 1950s.

Epidemic expansion to 1960

The Congo River and its tributaries link Cameroon with DRC and the Congo. Very likely someone with an early HIV-1 M group infection in Cameroon traveled downriver to DRC (which was at that time the Belgian Congo; this book uses place names in 2007, with occasional mention of historic names). HIV reached DRC very soon after the most recent common ancestor of the M group. We know this because the diversity in genetic sequences among M group viruses collected in DRC is comparable to the diversity found among all M group viruses from all over the world.

The earliest known HIV was found in one of approximately 700 blood samples collected from adults and children in various locations throughout DRC in 1959. The sample with HIV came from an adult male in Kinshasa.[8] Hundreds of kilometers away, in northern DRC, a woman was hospitalized in 1958 with 'swollen lymph nodes, breathing difficulties, and dental problems,'[9] and died in 1962 with what was later identified (from symptoms, without a confirming test for HIV infection) to be AIDS.[10] The earliest known O group infection was identified in a Norwegian sailor who visited Douala port in Cameroon in 1961-62. The sailor along with his wife and a child died from AIDS in 1976. Subsequent tests of stored tissues identified HIV-1 from the O group.[11]

The fact that we can identify three unlinked HIV-1 infections or AIDS cases from Africa around 1960 suggests that HIV infections were not rare. By the 1960s, the HIV-1 M and O groups had spread to many people. How many?

Intriguingly, doctors in Central Africa reported normally rare infections during 1930-60 which were later found to be common in people with AIDS. For example, Thijs reported more than 200 cases of Kaposi's sarcoma, a cancer caused by a virus, during 1939-55 in the DRC, along with other cases from Rwanda and Burundi.[12] In a substantial minority of these cases, Kaposi's sarcoma appeared in people aged less than 30 years, and infected lymph nodes and internal organs, a presentation that has later been associated with AIDS. (In people without AIDS, Kaposi's sarcoma is rare, and classically presents as infected patches of skin on the feet and legs of older men.) Doctors also reported cryptococcal meningitis and histoplasmosis, fungal infections later found to be common among people with AIDS.[13]

However, there is no consensus about whether any of these pre-1960 infections in Africa point to early AIDS cases.

Molecular clues to epidemic expansion

Viral sequences provide clues to early epidemic expansion. Most HIV-1 M group viruses can be sorted into one of nine subtypes or clades, which are identified by letters A through K (except E and I). The viruses in each of these clades are more closely related to each other – that is, their sequences are more similar – than to other HIV-1 M group viruses. The clades, in other words, are major limbs on the viral tree.

When one looks closely at HIV-1 sequences, many viruses are a mix of HIV-1 from two or more clades. These mixed viruses, or 'recombinants,' develop in people who have somehow acquired two or more HIV infections. Several dozen of these mixed viruses have spread to many people, establishing major branches on the viral tree. These common recombinants are called circulating recombinant forms, or CRFs. Most of the founder viruses for clades and CRFs can be dated to the 1950s or later.

Importantly, many HIV-1 M group viruses collected in Central Africa have no close relative among other viruses that have been sequenced – they cannot be assigned to any clade or CRF. In other words, these unclassified viruses identify a separate chain of infection (branch of the viral tree) going back to the early decades of the M group.

The Los Alamos National Laboratory in the US collects and posts sequences of HIV-1 molecules from studies throughout the world in the HIV Sequence Database.[14] As of October 2006, this Database listed over 100 unclassified HIV-1 M group samples from six countries in Central Africa. About 5 percent of samples were unclassified in DRC, 2 percent in Cameroon, and 3 percent in four other countries of the region (Central African Republic [CAR], Congo, Equatorial Guinea, and Gabon). Studies to date have sampled and sequenced HIV-1 from far less than 1 percent of Central Africans living with HIV-1 infections. If we could sequence HIV from all current infections, we would very likely find more than a thousand unclassified viruses descending from separate early branches (infections) in the first several decades of the epidemic.

There is also some evidence for early expansion in the HIV-1 O group. Relative to the M group, a larger proportion of O group sequences have no recent relatives. The O group viral tree, in other words, has many long branches – chains of infection – that began in the first several decades after the O group began to spread among humans. Current low numbers of HIV-1 O group infections – possibly 10,000 in the world – are evidence for long periods of slow growth,[15] no growth, or even declines in the number of infections. Analyses of available sequences cannot distinguish between these different possibilities, and so provide little information about the numbers of O group infections during 1920-60.

HIV-2 origin and epidemic expansion to 1960

Just as HIV-1 comes from chimpanzees and gorillas, HIV-2 comes from SIVs that passed from sooty mangabeys – which are native to West Africa – to humans. As of 2007, all known HIV-2s can be sorted into eight groups, labeled A through H. Each group appears to have begun with a separate transmission of SIV from sooty mangabeys to humans. Groups A and B account for most infections. Each of the other six groups, C through H, has been found in only one infection.

Molecular analyses have found that HIV-2 from the A and B groups is most closely related to SIV from sooty mangabeys in Cote d'Ivoire, suggesting that these groups began with SIV transmissions to humans in or near Cote d'Ivoire.[16] As of 2006, the one available estimate for the date of the most recent common ancestor of the HIV-2 A group is 1940. However, this is based on only 17 samples, of which at least 13 came from Guinea-Bissau (a Portuguese colony till 1974) or Portugal. Similarly, the one available estimate for the date of the last parent of all HIV-2 B group viruses – 1945 – is even more weakly based on only five samples.[17] Including more samples in these analyses will likely increase the range of sequence diversity, and thereby push the estimated dates of their most recent common ancestors back into the 1930s or earlier.

There is very little information to describe and date the spread of the HIV-2 A and B groups from Cote d'Ivoire and/or Liberia to other countries in West Africa. Rare cases of HIV-2 infection have been identified from stored blood samples collected in Cote d'Ivoire, Gabon, Mali, Nigeria, and Senegal in the period 1965-74.[18] The best source of information may be from sequencing, but so far not enough HIV-2s have been sequenced to get a picture of early epidemic spread.

Because people can live with HIV-2 infection for decades, even surviving to old age, surveys in the 1990s and even later provide information on HIV-2 prevalence in previous decades. Among countries, Guinea-Bissau has the highest HIV-2 prevalence and – based on infections in older persons[19] – may well have had the highest HIV-2 prevalence from before 1960.

Why did the HIV epidemic emerge in the 20th century?

As of 2007, sequencing of SIV and HIV has found 11 groups of HIV that descend from separate events in which SIV passed to a human – twice from chimpanzees, once from a gorilla, and eight times from sooty mangabeys. Recent studies in Central Africa report near matches between other bloodborne viruses (for example, simian foamy virus)[20] in humans and in simians, pointing to other recent simian-to-human transmissions. This evidence suggests that common events, such as a hunter or butcher getting simian blood into a cut, pass bloodborne viruses from simians to humans.

Because SIV passed from simians to humans at least 11 times in the recent past, this no doubt occurred in the distant past as well. SIV from chimpanzees – which started the HIV-1 M group – has been the most deadly for humans. Very likely SIV has passed from chimpanzees to humans hundreds of times in the more than 100,000 years during which humans lived near SIV-infected chimpanzees in Africa. In past centuries, no doubt some men and women with rare HIV infections from gorillas, chimpanzees, and sooty mangabeys sometimes transmitted HIV to others through wounds, scarification and other traditional skin-piercing practices, sex, or mother-to-child. But because the parent viruses for all HIV-1 and HIV-2 groups can be dated to the 20th century, we can conclude that – on average – each person infected with HIV before the 20th century infected less than one other person, so that rare infections did not multiply, but rather died out over time.

Hence, the puzzle that must be solved to explain the origin of the AIDS epidemic is not how SIV passed to humans, but what happened next, so that HIV passed from one human to another fast enough to survive and to spread among humans. This insight undermines explanations for the origins of the epidemic that focus on the particular time and route for SIV to pass from chimpanzees to humans.

Specifically, this insight undermines the hypothesis – articulated by Edward Hooper in *The River*[21] – that feeding of SIV-contaminated oral polio vaccine to 900,000 children and adults in Central Africa during 1957-60 caused the HIV epidemic. Even if contaminated vaccine had infected one or more persons, that alone would not explain the epidemic, because SIV had likely reached and infected humans many times in past millennia without starting an epidemic. There are other problems with this hypothesis. There is no solid evidence that the vaccine was prepared in chimpanzee kidney cells. There is no evidence it was contaminated with SIV. Even if the vaccine had been contaminated, HIV transmits poorly through oral exposures. And the hypothesized passage of SIV to humans through polio vaccine during 1957-60 occurred years after the estimated dates of the most recent common ancestors of the HIV-1 M and O groups.

What changed?

Three competing hypotheses attribute HIV's more successful human-to-human transmission in the period 1920-60 than in previous centuries to: more risky sex, more blood exposures, and viral evolution. More than one of these hypotheses could be at least partially true, and other factors – including so far unsuspected factors – may have also contributed to the early and unnoticed expansion of the HIV epidemic.

Hypothesis 1: More risky sex accelerated HIV transmission

This seems to be the most popular hypothesis, in line with the widespread assumption that sexual transmission drives Africa's HIV epidemics. Did Africans have more sexual partners during 1920-60 than in previous centuries? If so, did this accelerate HIV transmission enough to create an epidemic? The hypothesis is speculative at best, because there is so little information about sexual behavior in the decades and centuries before 1960.

Moreover, some evidence undercuts this hypothesis. As John Seale, an expert on sexually transmitted diseases, pointed out in 1987, 'Promiscuous sexual intercourse is not new in Africa, or in any other continent...'[22] Even so, there is no evidence that HIV survived before

1900 among Africans with frequent short-term sexual partners, such as warriors, long-distance traders, or women in sex work. If urbanization changed sexual behavior, then one would expect HIV to go to all cities in the region. But there were few HIV infections in Lagos or in other cities in Nigeria until after 1980.

Hence, the hypothesis that sexual behavior change was the primary factor accelerating HIV transmission in the early decades of the epidemic does not easily fit some evidence. However, considering the limited evidence, anything is possible.

Hypothesis 2: More blood exposures accelerated HIV transmission

In the mid-1980s, Seale proposed that 'medically promiscuous hypodermics' were responsible for the emergence of the HIV epidemic.[23] In 2000, Chitnis and co-authors identified 'medical campaigns against smallpox and sleeping sickness' in French colonies in Central Africa as possible factors in the origin of HIV.[24] Many others have suggested that blood exposures may have played a role.

Injection practices in Europe and the US before 1950

The first syringes with needles small enough to penetrate the skin are credited to Charles Pravaz of France and Alexander Wood of Scotland around 1850. Over time, doctors found more things to inject. Because of insufficient care taken to sterilize instruments between patients, injections exposed people to small amounts of blood – and bloodborne pathogens – from previous patients. This was an unprecedented challenge to human immune systems,[25] which had evolved with reliance on skin to prevent all but rare blood exposures.

In 1883-84, 191 of 1,350 workers at a German shipyard developed jaundice, a symptom of liver disease, after smallpox vaccination.[26] These were the first reported cases of jaundice linked to invasive healthcare. Through the 1940s, doctors in Europe and the US recognized jaundice – likely caused by hepatitis B virus infection – after a variety of invasive procedures including collecting blood and injecting gold salts and other drugs.[27]

In the first half of the 20th century – before penicillin – common treatment for syphilis entailed 15 or more weekly intravenous (into a vein) injections of arsenic compounds. In busy clinics, the usual practice was to change needles between patients, but to rinse and reuse syringes. For decades doctors wondered why so many patients treated for syphilis developed jaundice. Many doctors blamed the injected arsenic. Finally, during World War II, doctors working with British and US soldiers were able to show that jaundice was often caused by an (unseen) infectious agent in blood. In the worst single outbreak, 28,000 US soldiers developed jaundice after injections of yellow fever vaccine prepared from infected human sera.[28] Around the same time, 68 percent of men treated for syphilis in one clinic in the United Kingdom (UK) developed jaundice.[29]

In a classic 1943-45 study, Laird demonstrated that using a sterile syringe and needle for every injection prevented jaundice after treatment for syphilis. After introducing these procedures in a UK military clinic, he found only one case of post-treatment jaundice in 167 patients.[30] Other research reported in 1943 showed that rinsing syringes did not stop patient-to-patient transmission of bloodborne pathogens. To mimic common procedures during intravenous injections, researchers drew a small amount of contaminated blood into a syringe. Next, they rinsed the syringe – drawing in and expelling water – as may as six times. Even after six rinses, they found bacteria in expelled water. The study recommended '(t)he use of a freshly boiled syringe for each patient...'[31]

At the time, a common technique for administering intramuscular (into a muscle) injections, recommended by the UK's Medical Research Council in 1945, 'employs a separate sterile needle for each injection, but does not sterilize the syringe, which contains several doses of inoculum, between injections.'[32] Mid-century research showed this practice also spreads infections. In a study reported in 1950, researchers took syringes filled with a sterile solution, injected some of the solution into mice infected with *Streptococcus pneumoniae* (a bloodborne bacteria), changed the needles, and then injected healthy mice. In two experiments, 35 of 46 previously healthy mice contracted fatal streptococcus infections.[33] Changing needles is not enough to protect subsequent patients, because blood and pathogens reach syringes through suction when needles are removed from the syringes, through back pressure from tissues during injections, and through mixing and movement of fluid through needles.[34]

In Europe and the US, unsafe practices for injections and other invasive healthcare spread bloodborne pathogens on a prodigious scale during the first half of the 20ᵗʰ century. What happened in Africa?

Blood exposures in Central and West Africa, 1920-60

Due in part to tropical diseases that killed a large percentage of Europeans who ventured inland into Central and West Africa before 1900, Europeans did not claim control over much of the area until the late 19ᵗʰ century. Colonial rule ended in most countries of the region around 1960. Between these dates, colonial governments and missionaries extended European medical systems and techniques into Central and West Africa.

Throughout the African colonies of the imperialist nations, one of the most common invasive procedures was immunization against smallpox. In French colonies from the 1930s, and later in English colonies, health services injected BCG (Bacillus Calmette-Guerin) vaccine to prevent tuberculosis. Common invasive procedures in curative care included injections of quinine to treat malaria, and of arsenic-based drugs, bismuth, and later penicillin to cure yaws (most patients presented with persistent sores) and syphilis. After 1950, injected streptomycin treated tuberculosis.

Africans who traveled – such as civil servants, soldiers, and labor conscripts – were subject to more invasive procedures. In 1910, the Belgian Congo introduced medical passports.[35] French and Belgian colonial governments established filter posts along major transportation arteries to inspect travelers and their health documents. Health posts routinely detained and treated travelers before allowing them to proceed.

Long-running programs to control sleeping sickness, with frequent and repeated invasive procedures, may have been the most important public health programs for passage of bloodborne pathogens.

Sleeping sickness control programs in Central and West Africa

Two major variants of sleeping sickness, also known as human African trypanosomiasis, are caused by two subspecies of trypanosomes, a one-celled parasite. The two subspecies cannot be distinguished by their appearance under a microscope, but cause different patterns of infection and disease in humans and in other animals. The tsetse fly is an intermediate host, passing trypanosomes between humans and/or other animals.

One variant of the disease – the one which is important for this story – occurs in West and Central Africa. Europeans recognized sleeping sickness in small numbers of West Africans from the 18th century. In 1901, Forde and Dutton discovered trypanosomes – specifically, *Trypanosoma brucie*, subspecies *gambiense* – in the blood of a patient suffering from sleeping sickness in the Gambia.[36] This subspecies circulates primarily among humans. Some who are infected are lethargic, emaciated, and drowsy – symptoms which give the disease its name. Without treatment, such people die. However, many people infected with *T.b. gambiense* report no or only mild symptoms,[37] and no studies show how often and how fast untreated infections progress to debilitating illness.

Around 1900, the worst recorded epidemic of sleeping sickness erupted east of DRC in Uganda, at that time a British colony. During 1900-20, this epidemic killed an estimated 250,000 people – a third of the population – over 10,000 square kilometers along the north shore of Lake Victoria and extending inland. The British government organized a Sleeping Sickness Commission, which in 1903 identified trypanosomes as the cause of the epidemic.[38]

At that time and for many decades, most people thought that the trypanosomes that caused the Ugandan epidemic were from the subspecies *T.b. gambiense* that circulates in West and Central Africa. However, a recent review of the symptoms of those who died attributes the 1900-20 Ugandan epidemic to the subspecies *T.b. rhodesiense*,[39] which circulates among cattle and wild animals in East and Southern Africa. This subspecies occasionally infects humans, causing local epidemics with rapidly progressing and often fatal disease patterns.

The Ugandan epidemic motivated colonial governments in Central Africa to look for trypanosomes in their subjects. King Leopold of Belgium arranged for the Liverpool School of Tropical Medicine to send a team to DRC in 1903.[40] The Liverpool team reported as many as 30-50 percent of Africans infected with trypanosomes – presumably *T.b. gambiense* – in some villages along a particular river route, but this was unusual. In most communities, none or only a few percent of those they tested were infected.[41] Other surveys in West and Central Africa in the first several decades of the 20th century found trypanosomes in small (and rarely large) percentages of Africans in communities exposed to tsetse flies.

The French, Belgian, and German governments (Germany controlled Cameroon till 1914), fearing that these infections were the prelude to massive and deadly epidemics, took strong measures to protect their colonial populations. Initially, colonial governments sequestered hundreds of people found with trypanosomes into isolated settlements – often resembling prisons – to prevent tsetse flies from passing trypanosomes to others.

By 1906, European chemists had developed an injectable arsenic-based drug, atoxyl, that could eliminate trypanosomes from blood. Other drugs followed. With these drugs, doctors in French and Belgian colonies in Central and West Africa undertook the stupendous task of finding all people with trypanosomes – with or without symptoms – and injecting drugs to 'sterilize' their blood. The guiding goal was not to cure those who were infected, but to protect others by removing the risk that a biting fly might pick up and pass trypanosomes to them. Over time, drugs and treatment improved, so that people suffering from sleeping sickness – with symptoms, not just infections – more often recovered.

Eugene Jamot was an influential innovator and manager in French efforts to eliminate trypanosomes from African blood. In 1917-19, Jamot organized and led a team that toured parts of what is now CAR to find and treat people infected with trypanosomes.[42] The use of mobile teams for sleeping sickness control spread throughout Central and later West Africa. Visiting teams summoned all adults and children for inspection, at times relying on militia and on threats to collect people.[43] Doctors and assistants examined people for clinical signs of infection, such as swollen lymph glands in the side of the neck. Taking people with clinical signs, and sometimes without, mobile teams looked for trypanosomes in fluid aspirated (taken by syringe and needle) from lymph glands and/or in drops of blood from pricked fingers. Beginning in the 1920s, doctors routinely examined the cerebrospinal fluid, extracted by lumbar puncture, of all persons with confirmed or suspected infection.

Through 1932, health officials in Cameroon recorded more than 300,000 people – 12 percent of the population – with trypanosomes. Surveys in some communities in Cameroon in the late 1920s found trypanosomes in more than 50 percent of the population.[44] Doctors in French Equatorial Africa (currently CAR, Chad, Congo, and Gabon) found an average of roughly 10,000 new cases annually during 1921-1934.[45] In DRC, mobile teams visited at least a third of the population during most years from 1926 to 1945 and found a cumulative total of 360,000 persons – approximately 5 percent of the population – with trypanosomes.[46] In French West Africa (currently Benin, Burkina Faso, Cote d'Ivoire, Guinea, Mali, Mauritania, Niger, and Senegal), the annual number of new cases discovered ranged from 20,000-30,000 during 1934-42 (except 1939, when World War II disrupted sleeping sickness surveys).[47]

Drugs, treatment, and follow-up varied from place to place and over time. In 1928, standard treatment in Cameroon was a series of six subcutaneous (under the skin) injections of atoxyl or 10 intravenous injections of another arsenic-based drug.[48] Standard treatment in one part of DRC in 1931 was 40 injections administered on consecutive days.[49] After a course of injections, doctors repeated tests to assess the success of the treatment. For example, doctors in Kasai Province of DRC in the 1930s followed people for five years after treatment. Not until patients' cerebrospinal fluid was normal in five consecutive annual lumbar punctures were they considered to be cured.[50] If not, they received another series of injections, and so on. A review of 3,705 persons treated during 1919-1935 in CAR reported a total of 108,003 injections – an average of 29 per patient.[51] One unfortunate patient in DRC in the 1930s received 150 injections in less than five years, along with multiple lumbar punctures.[52]

Some of the common drugs caused temporary or even permanent damage to eyesight for several percent of persons treated. Around 1930, a doctor in Cameroon prescribed excessive doses that blinded more than 700 people.[53] Cameroon's colonial government held Jamot, the director of Cameroon's sleeping sickness program, to be responsible, and refused to allow him to return after a visit to France. Jamot moved to French West Africa, where he led sleeping sickness campaigns during 1932-35.

New trypanosome infections and treatment fell off from 1930 in Central Africa, and from the 1940s in West Africa. For example, in every year during 1937-45, surveys in DRC found new infections in less than 3 in 1,000 persons examined.[54] From the late 1940s, French and Belgian colonies in Central and West Africa introduced twice-yearly injections of diamidine for prophylaxis against infection by trypanosomes.[55] These injections concentrated in communities considered to have the greatest risk for sleeping sickness, which generally meant the same communities that had been most intensively treated to date.

Did programs to 'sterilize' African blood stop deadly epidemics, or were *T.b. gambiense* infections self-limiting in most individuals and in their communities? Nigeria, a British colony wedged between French colonies in West and Central Africa, arranged some sleeping sickness surveys, but these were not as extensive as in neighboring French colonies. In 1938, an official in Nigeria's Sleeping Sickness Service assessed: 'Taken as a whole the disease is of a mild type.' Most people found with trypanosomes had only intermittent symptoms, and had reached a stage where their 'disease and...resistance to it seem to have obtained a state of equilibrium.'[56] During surveys, 'Signs of nervous involvement were rare.' It was 'difficult to make the survey findings fit the classical picture.'[57]

Some recent evidence supports this less alarmist view of *T.b. gambiense* infections. A 2000-02 study of a suspected sleeping sickness outbreak in a community in DRC reported 77 people infected with trypanosomes, and attributed four deaths to sleeping sickness over three years – showing an average of just over one death per year against 77 infections.[58] The low ratio of deaths to infections could be explained by a sudden upsurge of infections and effective treatment on the one hand, or by a lot of chronic and non-progressing or defeated infections on the other. Despite all the efforts to control *T.b. gambiense*, the natural course of infection in humans is not yet well known.

Nosocomial transmission of hepatitis B and C viruses in Africa

In Africa, Jamot recommended boiling syringes and needles for at least 30 minutes, and changing needles for each patient.[59] Even if injectors followed these procedures, they would have routinely reused syringes without sterilization. In Europe and the US, similar practices before 1950 have been retrospectively credited with causing thousands of cases of post-treatment jaundice. What evidence is there that injections before 1960 spread bloodborne pathogens in Africa?

Aside from HIV, hepatitis B and C viruses are the most important bloodborne pathogens recognized to date. Both these viruses have circulated among humans in Africa for thousands of years.[60] However, the percentage of Africans infected with either of these viruses appears to have been low until at least 1850. The evidence for this is that there is much more genetic diversity among these viruses in Central and West Africa than in the Americas. This implies that the slave trade during 1500-1850 did not transport many infected Africans to the Americas, which in turn implies that low percentages of Africans were infected before 1850.

Not long after the hepatitis B virus was discovered in the 1960s, surveys found that 8-20 percent of African adults had active (mostly chronic) hepatitis B infections.[61] The implicit huge increase in hepatitis B infections among Africans after 1850 – if, indeed, that is what happened – could be explained by blood exposures during colonial and post-colonial healthcare. In contrast, only 0.2-0.5 percent of people in North America and Western Europe have active hepatitis B infections. (Chapters 3 and 8 consider the influential view that unsafe healthcare contributes little or nothing to Africa's hepatitis B problem.)

The hepatitis C virus was discovered in 1989. Just as for hepatitis B, prevalence of hepatitis C infection in Central and West Africa appears to have increased from low levels before 1850 to some of the highest levels in the world. Recent estimates show 13.8 percent of people in Cameroon infected with hepatitis C, 5.5 percent in DRC, and 9.2 percent in Gabon.[62] In contrast, in rich countries, the prevalence of hepatitis C infection seldom exceeds 2 percent, and most infections are from IDU or from transfusion of blood or blood products before reliable tests for the virus were introduced in the early 1990s. (Most estimates of the number of people with hepatitis C infections are based on tests for antibodies, not for the virus. Because some people with or without antibodies have defeated the virus, these estimates may overstate current infections, but may also miss many past and defeated infections.)

Infection with hepatitis C points to blood exposures. The virus seldom passes through vaginal or even anal sex, or from mother to child. For example, one study in Italy followed 776 couples in which one partner was infected. After 10 years, with an average of 1.8 coital acts per week, and no condom use – a total of 70,000 unprotected coital acts – not one spouse had acquired hepatitis C from their infected partner.[63]

23

Egypt has the highest estimated prevalence of hepatitis C infection – 18 per cent – in the world.[64] Egypt's high prevalence has been attributed to public health campaigns in the period 1961-86 to treat schistosomiasis (a parasite infection) with 12-16 intravenous injections.[65] Apparently, many of the injections were delivered with needles and/or syringes reused without sterilization.

In former French and Belgian colonies in Central Africa, several pieces of evidence suggest that high prevalence of hepatitis C infection can be traced to healthcare during colonial rule, and more specifically to programs to eradicate trypanosomes from the blood of Africans. Because most people infected with hepatitis C live normal lives – only a minority develops liver disease – one would expect to see a steady increase in infection with age. Older people, just by living longer, have had more blood exposures.

However, in Central Africa, and especially in Cameroon, much higher prevalence in persons born before 1960 suggests that rates of transmission of hepatitis C virus were high before 1960, and then fell sharply around 1960 and stayed low for decades.[66] For example, a survey in a rural forest area in southern Cameroon in 1990 found that 98 (33 per cent) of 298 persons over 40 years old – who were born before 1950 – carried antibodies to hepatitis C, compared to only three of 509 persons aged less than 40 years.[67] Rates of hepatitis C infection in older people in some communities are comparable to what is seen among IDUs, and are evidence for common and repeated blood exposures before 1960.

An analysis of genetic sequences from several hundred hepatitis C viruses collected in Cameroon concluded that the number of infections began to grow rapidly in 1920, and continued to do so up to 1960. This period of rapid growth 'coincided with the mass campaign against trypanosomiasis and mass vaccinations in Cameroon.'[68] The apparent slowing of hepatitis C transmission around 1960 coincides with the end of colonial rule – and a cut-back in sleeping sickness surveys and injections.

In addition, the geographic distribution of hepatitis C infections shows parallels with the distribution of sleeping sickness interventions. At the country level, the prevalence of hepatitis C infection is greater in former French colonies (for example, 13.8 percent in Cameroon) than in adjacent former British colonies (for example, 2.1 percent in Nigeria),[69] where authorities paid less attention to the disease. Within Cameroon, higher prevalence of hepatitis C infection is found in communities more exposed to tsetse flies, where people were more likely to carry trypanosomes, and thus more likely to receive injections to 'sterilize' their blood. For example, one study found that prevalence of hepatitis C antibodies was three times greater in villages surrounded by forests – where villagers were exposed to flies from the forest – than in villages surrounded by fields.[70]

Evidence suggesting that healthcare transmitted HIV

The best estimates for the time and place for the origin of the HIV-1 O and M groups are in Cameroon in the several decades before 1940, when colonial healthcare workers identified and treated more than 300,000 people infected with trypanosomes. In DRC, healthcare programs administered millions of invasive procedures to control sleeping sickness and other diseases during 1930-60 when the HIV-1 M group multiplied and spread. Similarly, SIV apparently passed from sooty mangabeys to begin the HIV-2 A and B groups in or near Cote d'Ivoire. Through 1945, sleeping sickness surveillance found more than 46,000 people infected with trypanosomes in Cote d'Ivoire.[71] These coincidences do not prove causation, but they allow it.

Because people can live for many years with HIV-2 infections, a study in 2005 among people aged 50 years and older in Guinea-Bissau has been able to identify long-ago blood exposures – some of which occurred before 1960 – as risks for HIV-2 infection. Over half of those tested were aged over 60 years, and therefore born before 1945. People with HIV-2 were more likely than people without HIV-2 to have received injections to treat tuberculosis or sleeping sickness (the peak in sleeping sickness diagnoses in Guinea-Bissau occurred in the early 1950s). Women with HIV-2 infections were more likely to have been circumcised (female circumcision was commonly performed on groups of girls aged 8-12 years). The study team concluded that HIV-2[72]

> spread parenterally [though blood exposures] starting in the late 1940s, through needles, syringes, and instruments used for excision... We documented three routes for parenteral transmission, but it is possible that others existed.

People infected with HIV-1 characteristically have much more virus per cubic centimeter of blood than do people infected with HIV-2. Thus, wherever HIV-1 was available, invasive procedures similar to those that transmitted HIV-2 in Guinea-Bissau likely passed HIV-1 from person-to-person. High prevalence of hepatitis C infection in Central Africa attests to frequent blood exposures during 1920-60. Because HIV-1 was present during much of that time, blood exposures likely spread HIV-1 as well.

Intriguingly, the evident drop in hepatitis C transmission in Cameroon and in other former French colonies in Central Africa around 1960 may point to a temporary reduction in bloodborne transmission of HIV as well. If so, this could help to explain the low prevalence of HIV infection found in Cameroon in the early 1980s.

Hypothesis 3: More blood exposures allowed HIV to adapt to humans

One variant of the hypothesis that invasive healthcare in Africa accounts for the emergence of HIV epidemics in the 20th century supposes that it allowed HIV to evolve.[73] According to this hypothesis, the transmission of SIV from a simian to a human leads to an infection that the human can suppress or even eliminate within weeks to months. The hypothesis goes on to propose that blood exposures during healthcare in the 20th century transmitted a rare and fleeting HIV infection through several people, and that this 'serial passaging' of HIV though one person after another allowed the virus to live and multiply in humans long enough to evolve. Having adapted to humans, it could maintain sustained infections, and could transmit more easily from one human to another. Serial passaging could have occurred through invasive healthcare in French and Belgian colonies before World War II.[74]

But was serial passaging necessary? If unsterile invasive procedures were sufficiently common to passage several rare, unadapted HIVs from cut hunters or butchers through 3-4 people in a year, that same frequency of unsterile procedures could spread HIV from one infection to thousands over several decades. To create the HIV epidemic, there would be no need to hypothesize evolutionary change in HIV.

The hypothesis assumes that SIV from chimpanzees would have difficulty living in humans. But many viruses survive and spread after cross-species transmission. HIV has no doubt evolved in humans over time, but the evidence to date does not show that change in HIV (as against change in people's sexual and/or medical practices) was the key that allowed HIV to spread among humans.

Unrecognized risks

During the colonial era, which ended for most Africans around 1960, a lot of evidence suggests that blood exposures during healthcare spread bloodborne viruses. At least until 1950, most doctors were not aware of how easy it was to transmit infections through instruments reused without sterilization. Hence, much of the damage could be attributed to hubris – doctors thinking they knew more than they did, and thus subjecting patients to unknown risks.

Colonial healthcare programs in Central and West Africa no doubt transmitted HIV along with other bloodborne pathogens. But was this a minor or a major contributor to the emergence of HIV-1 and HIV-2 epidemics? More information from sequencing – especially if old HIV can be sequenced from stored blood – and from other sources may advance our understanding of the early epidemic, and could change current views, as described in this chapter.

---

[1] Switzer WM, Parekh B, Shanmugam V, et al. 'The epidemiology of simian immunodeficiency virus infection in a large number of wild- and captive-born chimpanzees: Evidence for a recent introduction following chimpanzee divergence', *AIDS Res Hum Retroviruses*, 2005, 21: 335-42.

[2] Keele BF, Van Heuverswyn F, Li Y, et al. 'Chimpanzee reservoirs of pandemic and nonpandemic HIV-1', *Science*, 2006, 313: 523-6.

[3] Van Heuverswyn F, Li Y, Neel C, et al. 'SIV infection in wild gorillas', *Nature*, 2006, 444: 164.

[4] Yusim K, Peeters M, Pybus OG, et al. 'Using human immunodeficiency virus type 1 sequences to infer historical features of the acquired immune deficiency syndrome epidemic and human immunodeficiency virus evolution', *Phil Trans R Soc Lond B*, 2001, 356: 855-66; Korber B, Muldoon M, Theiler J, et al. 'Timing the ancestor of the HIV-1 pandemic strains', *Science* 2000; 288; 1789-96; Salemi M, Strimmer K, Hall WW, et al. 'Dating the common ancestor of SIVcpz and HIV-1 M group and the origin of the HIV-1 sub-types by using a new method to uncover clock-like molecular evolution', *FASEB J*, 2001; 15: 276-8.

[5] Roques P, Robertson DL, Souquiere S, et al. 'Phylogenetic analysis of 49 newly derived HIV-1 group O strains: high viral diversity but no group M-like subtype structure', *Virology*, 2002, 302: 259-73.

[6] Lemey P, Pybus OG, Rambaut A, et al. 'The molecular population genetics of HIV-1 group O', *Genetics*, 2004, 167: 1059-68.

[7] Roques P, Robertson DL, Souquiere S, et al. 'Phylogenetic characteristics of three new HIV-1 N strains and implications for the origin of group N', *AIDS*, 2004, 18: 1371-81.

[8] Zhu T, Korber BT, Nahmias AJ, et al. 'An African HIV-1 sequence from 1959 and implications for the origin of the epidemic', *Nature*, 1998, 391: 594-7; Motulsky AG, Vandepitte J, Fraser GR. 'Population genetic studies in the Congo: I. Glucose-6-phosphate dehydrogenase deficiency, hemoglobin S and malaria', *Am J Hum Genet*, 1966, 18: 514-37.

[9] Hooper E. *The River*. London: Penguin, 2000. p. 260.

[10] Sonnet J, Michaux J-L, Zech F, et al. 'Early AIDS cases originating from Zaire and Burundi (1962-1976)', *Scand J Infect Dis*, 1987, 19: 511-17.

[11] Vangroenweghe D. 'The earliest cases of human immunodeficiency virus type 1 group M in Congo-Kinshasa, Rwanda and Burundi and the origin of acquired immune deficiency syndrome', *Phil Trans R Soc Lond B*, 2001, 356: 923-5; Jonassen TO, Stene-Johansen K, Berg ES, et al. 'Sequence analysis of HIV-1 group O from Norwegian patients infected in the 1960s', *Virology*, 1997, 231: 43-7.

[12] Thijs A. 'L'angiosarcomatose de Kaposi au Congo belge et au Ruanda-Urundi', *Ann Soc Belge Med Trop*, 1957, 37: 295-305.

[13] Molez J-F. 'The historical question of acquired immunodeficiency syndrome in the 1960s in the Congo River basin area in relation to cryptococcal meningitis', *Am J Trop Med Hyg*, 1998, 58: 273-6; Devreese A, Donkers J, Ninane G, et al. 'Histoplasmose africaine a formes capsulatum causee par Histoplasma dubosii Vanbreuseghem 1952', *Ann Soc Belge Med Trop*, 1961, 5: 403-14.

[14] Los Alamos National Laboratory. *HIV Sequence Database*. Available at: http://www.hiv.lanl.gov/content/hiv-db (accessed 28 September 2006).

[15] Lemey P et al. 'The molecular population genetics of HIV-1 group O'.

[16] Santiago ML, Range F, Keele BF, et al. 'Simian immunodeficiency virus infection in free-ranging sooty mangebeys (*Cercocebus atys atys*) from the Tai Forest, Cote d'Ivoire: implications for the origin of endemic human immunodeficiency virus type 2', *J Virol*, 2005, 79: 12515-27.

[17] Lemey P, Pybus OG, Wang B, et al. 'Tracing the origin and history of the HIV-2 epidemic', *Proc Nat Acad Sci USA*, 2003, 100: 6588-92; Personal communication from Philippe Lemey, 28 September 2006.

[18] Kawamura M, Yamazaki S, Ishikawa K, et al. 'HIV-2 in West Africa in 1966 [letter]', *Lancet*, 1989, i: 385; Le Guenno B. 'HIV1 and HIV2: Two ancient viruses for a new disease', *Trans Roy Soc Trop Med Hygiene*, 1989, 83: 847.

[19] Wilkins A, Ricard D, Todd J, et al. 'The epidemiology of HIV infection in a rural area of Guinea-Bissau', *AIDS*, 1993, 7: 1119-22; Piedade J, Venenno T, Prieto E, et al. 'Longstanding presence of HIV-2 infection in Guinea-Bissau (West Africa)', *Acta Trop*, 2000, 76: 119-24; Pepin J, Plamondon M, Alves AC, et al. 'Parenteral transmission during excision and treatment of tuberculosis and trypanosomiasis may be responsible for the HIV-2 epidemic in Guinea-Bissau', *AIDS*, 2006, 20: 1303-11.

[20] Wolfe ND, Switzer WM, Carr JK, et al. 'Naturally acquired simian retrovirus infections in central African hunters', *Lancet*, 2004, 363: 932-7.

[21] Hooper E. *The River*.

[22] Seale JR, Medvedev ZA. 'Origin and transmission of AIDS. Multi-use hypodermics and the threat to the Soviet Union: Discussion paper', *J Roy Soc Med*, 1987, 80: 301-4. p. 302.

[23] Ibid., p. 302.

[24] Chitnis A, Rawls D, Moore J. 'Origin of HIV type 1 in colonial French Equatorial Africa?' *AIDS Res Hum Retroviruses*, 2000, 16: 5-8. p. 7.

[25] Drucker E, Alcabes PG, Marx PA. 'The injection century: Massive unsterile injections and the emergence of human pathogens', *Lancet*, 2001, 358: 1989-92.

[26] Dull HB, 'Syringe-transmitted hepatitis: A recent epidemic in historical perspective', *JAMA*, 1961, 176: 413-8.

[27] Laird SM. 'Syringe-transmitted hepatitis', *Glasgow Med J*, 1947, 28: 199-219.

[28] 'Jaundice following yellow fever vaccination', *JAMA*, 1942, 119: 1110.

[29] Salaman MH, King AJ, Williams DI, et al. 'Prevention of jaundice resulting from antisyphilitic treatment', *Lancet*, 1944, ii: 7-8.

[30] Laird SM. 'Syringe-transmitted hepatitis'.

[31] Bigger JW. 'Jaundice in syphilitics under treatment', *Lancet*, 1943: i: 457-8. p. 458.

[32] Evans RJ, Spooner ETC. A possible mode of transfer of infection by syringes used for mass inoculation. *Br Med J*, 1950, ii: 185-8. p. 185.

[33] Ibid.

[34] Hughes RR, Post-penicillin jaundice, *Br Med J*, 1946, 2: 685-8.

[35] Lyons M. *The Colonial Disease: A social history of sleeping sickness in northern Zaire, 1900-1940*. Cambridge: Cambridge University Press, 1992.

[36] Boyce R, Ross R, Sherrington CS. 'Note on the discovery of the human trypanosome [letter]', *Brit Med J*, 1902, 2: 1680.

[37] Lester HMO. 'Further progress in the control of sleeping sickness in Nigeria', *Trans Roy Soc Trop Med Hygiene*, 1945, 38: 425-44.

[38] Christy C. 'Sleeping sickness', *Journal of the Royal African Society*, 1903, 9(3): 1-11; Low GL. 'A retrospect of tropical medicine from 1894 to 1914', *Trans R Soc Trop Med Hyg*, 1929, 23: 213-34; Maudlin I. 'African trypanosomiasis', *Ann Trop Med Parasitology*, 2006, 100: 679-701.

[39] Fevre EM, Coleman PG, Welburn SC, et al. 'Reanalyzing the 1900-1920 sleeping sickness epidemic in Uganda', *Emerg Infect Dis*, 2004, 10: 567-73.

[40] Lyons M. 'From 'death camps' to condon sanitaire: the development of sleeping sickness policy in the Uele district of the Belgian Congo, 1903-1914', *Journal of African History*, 1985, 26: 69-91.

[41] Dutton JE, Todd JL. 'Distribution and spread of sleeping sickness in the Congo Free State', in: Dutton JE, Todd JL. *Reports of the Expedition to the Congo, 1903-5, Liverpool School of Tropical Medicine – Memoir XVIII*. London: Williams & Norgate, 1906. pp 23-38.

[42] Richet P. 'Eugene Jamot: Son oeuvre', *Med Trop* 1979; 39: 487-93.

[43] Headrick R. *Colonialism, Health and Illness in French Equatorial Africa, 1885-1935* (Headrick DR, ed). Atlanta: Africa Studies Association, 1994.

[44] Jamot E. 'La maladie du sommeil au Cameroun en janvier 1929', *Bull Soc Pathol Exot*,1929; 22: 473-96.

[45] Headrick R. *Colonialism, Health and Illness*.

[46] Van Hoof LMJJ. 'Observations on trypanosomiasis in the Belgian Congo', *Trans R Soc Trop Med Hyg*, 1947, 40: 728-61.

[47] Masseguin A, Taillefer-Grimaldi J. 'Declin et danger residuel de la trypanosomiase en Africque Occidentale Francaise', *Ann Soc Belg Med Trop*, 1954, 34: 671-96.

[48] Hermant I. 'Les maladies transmissibles observees dan les colonies francaises et territories sous mandate pendant l'annee 1928', *Ann Med Pharmacie Coloniales*, 1931, 29: 5-138.

[49] Lyons M. *The Colonial Disease*. p. 152.

[50] Haveaux G. 'Vingt ans d'action medicale contre la maladie du someil dans le Kasai', *Ann Soc Belge Med Trop*, 1945, 25: 155-203.

[51] Vamos S. 'Traitment de trypansomes dans un secteur du Moyen-Chari (A.E.F.) etude de 3,705 observations', *Bull Soc Pathol Exot*, 1936, 29: 1015-22.

[52] Van Hoof L, Henrard C, Peel E. 'Contribution a l'epidemiologie de la maladie du sommeil au Congo Belge', *Ann Soc Belge Med Trop*, 1938, 18: 143-201.

[53] Sanner L. 'Eugene Jamot: L'homme (1879-1937)', *Med Trop*, 1979, 39: 479-84.

[54] Van Hoof LMJJ. 'Observations on trypanosomiasis'.

[55] Lotte A. 'Enseigment de quatre annees de chimio-prophylaxie en A.E.F.', *Med Trop* 1951, 11: 737-66; Deroover J. 'Modifications de l'aspect de la trypanosomiase humaine a *Tr. gambianse* dans un vieux foyer, sous l'influence des methods modernes de prophylaxis et de therapeutique', *Ann Soc Belge Med Trop Trop*, 1958, 38: 149-78.

[56] Lester HMO. 'The progress of sleeping sickness work in northern Nigeria', *West Afr Med J*, 1938, 10: 2-10. p. 2.

[57] Lester HMO. 'Further progress'. p. 426.

[58] Lutumba P, Makieya E, Shaw A, et al. 'Human African trypanosomiasis in a rural community, Democratic Republic of Congo', *Emerg Infect Dis*, 2007, 13: 248-54.

[59] Jamot E. 'La maladie du sommeil'.

[60] Simmonds P. 'Reconstructing the origins of human hepatitis viruses', *Phil Trans R Soc Lond B 2001*, 356: 1013-26.

[61] Kiire CF. 'The epidemiology and control of hepatitis B in sub-Saharan Africa', *Prog Med Virol*, 1993, 40: 141-56; WHO. *Hepatitis B*. Geneva: WHO, 2002. Doc. no: WHO/CDS/CSR/LYO/2002.2:Hepatitis B.

[62] Madhava V, Burgess C, Drucker E. 'Epidemiology of chronic hepatitis C virus infection in sub-Saharan Africa', *Lancet Infect Dis*, 2002, 2: 293-302.

[63] Vandelli C, Renzo F, Romano L, et al. 'Lack of evidence of sexual transmission of hepatitis C among monogamous couples: Results of a 10-year prospective follow-up study', *Am J Gastroenterol*, 2004, 99: 855-9.

[64] 'Hepatitis C – Global prevalence (update)', *Wkly Epidemiol Rec*, 1999; 74: 425-7.

[65] Frank C, Mohamed MK, Strickland GT, et al. 'The role of parenteral antischistomal therapy in the spread of hepatitis C virus in Egypt', *Lancet*, 2000, 355: 887-91.

[66] Nerrienet E, Pouillot R, Lachenal G, et al. 'Hepatitis C virus infection in Cameroon: A cohort effect', *J Med Virol*, 2005, 76: 208-14.

[67] Louis FJ, Maubert B, Le Hesran JY, et al. 'High prevalence of anti-hepatitis C virus antibodies in a Cameroon rural forest area', *Trans R Soc Trop Med Hyg*, 1994, 88: 53-4.

[68] Njouom R, Nerrienet E, Dubois M, et al. 'The hepatitis C virus epidemic in Cameroon: genetic evidence for rapid transmission between 1920 and 1960', *Infect Genet Evol*, 2007, 7: 361-7. p. 361.

[69] Madhava V, Burgess C, Drucker E. 'Epidemiology of chronic hepatitis C virus infection'.

[70] Louis FJ, Kemmenge J. 'Grande variations de la prevalence de l'infection par le virus C des hepatites en Afrique centrale [letter]', *Med Trop*, 1994; 54: 277-8.

[71] Masseguin A, Taillefer-Grimaldi J. 'Declin et danger residuel de la trypanosomiase en Africque Occidentale Francaise', *Ann Soc Belg Med Trop*, 1954, 34: 671-96.

[72] Pepin J et al. 'Parenteral transmission', p. 1309.

[73] Marx P, Alcabes PG, Drucker E. 'Serial human passage of simian immunodeficiency virus by unsterile injections and the emergence of epidemic human immunodeficiency virus in Africa', *Phil Trans R Soc Lond B*. 2001, 356: 911-20.

[74] Moore J. 'The puzzling origins of AIDS', *Am Sci*, 2004, 92: 540-7.

Chapter 3

AIDS SPREADS SILENTLY, 1960-81

During 1960-81, the HIV epidemic expanded geographically, reaching more countries in Africa and also in the Americas and Europe. In parts of Central Africa, the epidemic grew slowly if at all. Infections multiplied much faster in some of the countries with newer epidemics both in and outside Africa.

Although sleeping sickness control programs contracted with the end of colonial rule, blood exposures throughout Africa generally increased with expanding foreign and multilateral aid, national health systems, and private healthcare. The contribution of HIV transmission through blood exposures to Africa's epidemic during this period remains a matter for speculation and investigation.

HIV-1 expansion in Africa, 1960-81

The HIV-1 M group apparently began with SIV passing from a chimpanzee to a human in southeast Cameroon. Low HIV prevalence in Cameroon at the beginning of the 1980s testifies to decades of slow or no epidemic expansion in that country. During 1960-81, the most intense epidemics in Africa developed in DRC and in DRC's neighbors to the north, east, and south.

More than 24,000 stored blood samples collected in Africa before 1982 have been tested for HIV.[1] From these samples, the highest rates of HIV-1 prevalence have been found in DRC and Burundi. In Kinshasa, tests of stored blood found 0.25 percent of 'healthy mothers' to be HIV-positive in 1970, increasing to 3 percent in 1980.[2] Tests of stored blood collected in 1976 from rural children and adults in north-central DRC found 0.8 percent to be HIV-positive (the blood was collected after an outbreak of Ebola hemorrhagic fever, which is discussed later in this chapter).[3] In Burundi, testing of blood samples collected in 1980-81 from a 'healthy population' including some children found 8.1 percent HIV prevalence in urban areas and 2.8 percent in selected rural areas (these and other results from stored blood are based on too few samples to give more than a rough idea about HIV prevalence before 1981).[4]

Most of the pre-1980 HIV infections and suspected AIDS deaths in Europeans linked to Africa have been traced to DRC, Rwanda, and Burundi in the 1960s and 1970s.[5] During 1960-81, doctors in DRC and in neighboring countries reported unusual numbers of patients with cryptococcal meningitis[6] and Kaposi's sarcoma (including some with infected lymph nodes, and some children). After 1981, these conditions have been associated with AIDS. Tests of blood collected in Kinshasa in 1972 from four patients with Kaposi's sarcoma found that two were HIV-positive.[7] Experts disagree about how often pre-1980 cases of Kaposi's sarcoma in Africans were associated with AIDS.

When HIV testing began in the mid-1980s, some of the highest rates of HIV prevalence were found in Rwanda and in communities west of Lake Victoria in northwest Tanzania and southwest Uganda. Unfortunately, not much information is available from tests of stored blood on pre-1980s HIV infections in those regions. Hooper in *The River* reports Kaposi's sarcoma and other often AIDS-related infections during the 1960s in immigrants from Rwanda and Burundi in Uganda.[8] A 1974 study reports 'a definite concentration of cases [of Kaposi's sarcoma] in western Uganda...which seems...to extend into Tanzania to the west and south of Lake Victoria and possibly across Rwanda and Burundi into the eastern [DRC].'[9]

Hooper speculates that refugees fleeing genocide in Rwanda around 1960 brought HIV to Tanzania and Uganda,[10] but there was a lot of normal cross-border traffic which could have done so as well. When I visited northwest Tanzania in 2000, a Canadian missionary told me that when he arrived in the early 1970s, people already recognized what they called slim disease, which was later found to be AIDS.

Before 1981, HIV had very likely passed south from DRC into Zambia, but there is no information from stored blood to show when HIV began to circulate in Zambia. In Zimbabwe, tests of several hundred blood samples from around 1970 found no HIV infections. HIV-1 no doubt reached West Africa before 1981, but infections were rare. Tests of more than 4,000 blood samples collected in West Africa in the 1960s and 1970s found no confirmed HIV-1 infections.[11]

Molecular evidence

The epidemic in DRC appears to have grown over time, rather than with a concentrated late growth spurt. The evidence for this is that

33

DRC's HIV epidemic established new major branches, such as clades, sub-clades (or sub-subtypes) and CRFs, progressively over time.[12] All clades in the HIV-1 M group began to multiply from parent (founder) viruses in or near DRC (except for clade B, for which the founder virus appears to have reached Haiti before multiplying). All clades, with a few possible exceptions, circulate across DRC and all former French colonies in Central Africa (Cameroon, CAR, Congo, Chad, and Gabon). However, the percentage of HIV infections from each clade varies across the region. For example, the C clade is more common in several southern cities in DRC than in north DRC.[13]

On the other hand, HIV-1 samples from African countries east and south of DRC and in West Africa show less clade diversity, pointing to rapid expansion from single viruses and/or multiple introductions of closely related viruses that have subsequently dominated the epidemics in those countries. For example, the C clade, which has been estimated to begin in the mid- to late 1960s,[14] appears to account for most infections in Burundi[15] and Zambia.[16]

Sex exposures in Africa

Many AIDS experts suppose that urbanization and other social changes in Africa during this period accelerated heterosexual transmission of HIV. According to Chin,[17]

> During the 1960s, concomitant with the attainment of independence for some African states, there were significant political and social upheavals, along with major movements of young adults, mostly males, to the growing urban centers in SSA [sub-Saharan Africa]. These population changes increased the introduction of HIV infections from relatively stable rural societies to the newly expanding urban centers where a more open and liberal social/sexual environment fostered the transmission of HIV. The patterns and high prevalence of heterosexual HIV risk behaviors in many SSA cities provided the fertile environment for HIV epidemic spread.

This picture fits some evidence. By 1980 at least 25 percent of the residents of Cameroon, CAR, Congo, DRC, Gabon, and Nigeria lived in cities.[18] Adult HIV prevalence had reached several percent in Kinshasa by 1980, and HIV was circulating across the river in Brazzaville (the capital of Congo), in Bangui (the capital of CAR), and no doubt also in other urban areas in DRC.

On the other hand, two of the three largest cities in the region were in Nigeria, with almost no HIV through the early 1980s. Moreover, African countries where HIV 'sparks' found the driest tinder during 1960-81 were not consistently distinguished by urban agglomerations or sexual behavior. Although only 4 percent of Burundians lived in cities in 1980, the country appears to have had one of the worst HIV epidemics at the beginning of the 1980s.

As noted above, the C clade, whose founder virus has been dated to the mid- to late 1960s, accounts for most HIV infections in Burundi. Thus Burundi's epidemic must have grown faster during the 1970s than older epidemics in Cameroon, Gabon, DRC, Congo, and CAR. However, sexual behavior in Burundi is relatively conservative. In a 1990 survey among urban Burundian adults aged 15-49 years, only 10 percent of men and 3 percent of women reported sex with a non-regular partner in the past 12 months. This was far less than percentages reporting non-regular sex partners in seven of eight other African countries with comparable surveys.[19]

In contrast, HIV prevalence among adults in Yaounde, the capital of Cameroon, the country with the world's oldest HIV-1 epidemic, was 0.3 percent only when this was first measured in 1987.[20] Conservative sexual behavior does not explain Yaounde's low HIV prevalence. In a 1997-98 survey, 67 percent of men and 44 percent of women in Yaounde reported one or more non-regular sex partners in the past 12 months.[21]

Blood exposures in Africa

When regional countries gained independence around 1960, new governments cut back or dismantled sleeping sickness control programs, perceiving them to be too expensive for so few infections.[22] However, expansion of other healthcare activities increased blood exposures over much of Africa. National governments and donors continued to channel a lot of resources through mobile teams and special programs, but over time shifted more efforts into hospitals and clinics. In addition, private formal and informal providers administered injections and other invasive procedures.

Mobile teams and special programs

From 1949, WHO promoted mobile teams to treat yaws, a disease characterized by troublesome sores and sometimes disfiguring damage to bones and cartilage. During 1950-66, yaws treatment programs administered one or more injections of long-acting penicillin to 20 million Africans[23] – at that time, approximately 1 in 12 Africans.

In 1967, WHO launched an Intensified Smallpox Eradication Program. The program used mobile teams to vaccinate people and to survey for cases. Depending on the country, these teams often provided BCG vaccinations (against tuberculosis) and/or other health care inspections and treatments as well. In Central, West, and East Africa, the number of smallpox vaccinations by country during the program generally exceeded the population, as some people were vaccinated more than once. The program identified the last naturally occurring smallpox infection in Somalia in 1977. Smallpox has been eradicated, except for frozen samples of the virus retained in several laboratories.

The Smallpox Eradication Program used bifurcated needles (with a split tip) to place a drop of vaccine on the skin, and to administer shallow jabs to get the vaccine under the skin. Instructions to vaccinators prescribed sterilization of needles between clients by boiling or flaming. For flaming, which was common, the instructions read: 'the needle is passed through the flame of a spirit lamp. It should not remain in the flame for more than three seconds.'[24] This upper time limit was set to prolong the life of the needle. Notably, the instructions did not prescribe a minimum time required to sterilize the needle. After flaming and cooling, the vaccinator dipped the needle in vaccine to pick up a drop for the next client. To contain costs, program managers pushed staff to vaccinate more people per day. Staff in Africa commonly vaccinated over 500 people per day. During one month in Rwanda the average was over 1,500 vaccinations per day per vaccinator.[25]

For other vaccines, health staff commonly changed needles between clients but reused syringes without sterilization. For example, a description of BCG vaccination in Sudan around 1970 reports that 'needles had to be flamed after each inoculation and the syringes repeatedly refilled from the vaccine vial.'[26] At the time, changing needles and reusing syringes remained common in the UK. As late as

1978 doctors in the UK injected children with BCG 'using a separate syringe for every 10 injections and a new needle for each child.'[27]

From 1974, WHO launched the Expanded Program on Immunization (EPI), which promoted immunizing children throughout the world against six diseases (tetanus, tuberculosis, polio, diphtheria, whooping cough, and measles), and immunizing women against tetanus, both to protect them during childbirth, and to protect their children from neo-natal tetanus. Before EPI, BCG vaccination was common in much of Africa, but coverage of the other vaccines was limited. In Africa, the program took time to get started, so that almost all the expansion in immunization coverage under EPI occurred in the 1980s and later.

Hospitals, clinics, and other healthcare providers

During 1950-70, governments and donors put a lot of effort into expanding Africa's hospitals. Whereas population grew by about 60 percent over these two decades, the number of hospital beds almost doubled. Thereafter, hospital expansion slowed. In the 1970s, public health experts increasingly recognized that Africa's hospitals absorbed an inordinate share of health budgets, and did not reach healthcare services to rural people. This realization led to a shift of emphasis towards primary healthcare delivered through local clinics.[28] In 1978, most governments in the world took part in the International Conference on Primary Health Care in Alma Ata, Kazakhstan. The conference declaration asked governments 'to launch and sustain primary health care as part of a comprehensive national health system,' promoted immunizations and maternal and child healthcare, and asked donors to give more money.[29]

As African medical schools produced more doctors, an increasing number went into private practice, opening their own clinics. In addition, pharmacists, traditional practitioners, and people with little or no training offered injections and other invasive healthcare in formal and informal settings. Because medical equipment – including syringes and needles – and injectable drugs were widely available without prescription, virtually anyone could provide an injection.[30]

Due in part to the dramatic cures seen with injections against yaws and other diseases, injections were popular.[31] Patients often expected or even demanded injections. During this time, common treatment for tuberculosis was 60 daily injections of streptomycin, and common treatment for syphilis was 10 daily injections of short-acting penicillin.

Unsterile practices were common, even in hospitals and clinics under foreign management. For example, a doctor in DRC reported in 1953 that the country[32]

> is strewn with various medical facilities – maternity clinics, hospitals, dispensaries – where local health care staff daily administer dozens and even hundreds of injections in conditions which make it impossible to sterilize the syringe or needle after each use. At the Red Cross clinic to treat sexually transmitted disease in Leopoldville [Kinshasa] around 300 injections are given each day...The used syringes are simply rinsed, first in water, then in alcohol and ether, and are then ready for reuse...Syringes pass therefore from one patient to another, conserving, sometimes, small quantities of contagious blood...

During the 1970s, recognized health consequences from reusing instruments without sterilization included bacterial abscesses, viral diseases, and tetanus. In Yaounde's Central Hospital in 1974-75, '14% of the tetanus cases reviewed...had an identifiable iatrogenic source of infection.'[33]

Some authors link an increase in reuse of syringes without sterilization during 1950-80 to the spread of plastic syringes intended for single use.[34] Because the high temperatures required for sterilization damaged or destroyed plastic syringes, they were often reused without sterilization. However, reuse without sterilization was common with glass syringes as well, both before and after plastic syringes came into common use.

Blood transfusions

Although blood transfusions can save lives, blood has always been dangerous to use, with known as well as unknown risks (such as unknown viruses). During the early 20th century, doctors learned how to overcome some of the short-term dangers due to mismatched blood types and clotting. Blood transfusions became common in rich countries before World War II. In Central Africa, transfusions were available from at least one site in DRC by 1924.[35]

The expansion and development of transfusion services to treat soldiers during World War II led to large post-war increases in the frequency of transfusions in Africa as well as in Europe and the US. Transfusion services expanded to at least 19 countries in Africa by 1955. The number of transfusions administered per decade in Africa (except South Africa and North Africa) has been estimated at 680,000 in the 1940s, increasing to 1.4 million in the 1950s, 5.2 million in the 1960s, and 12 million in the 1970s.[36] Doctors administered transfusions to treat not only people with acute blood loss, but also people with chronic anemia, such as from parasite infection. In addition, doctors used blood transfusions (convalescent serum) to treat people with infectious disease, injecting blood from someone who had recovered from the disease.

Blood transfusion was not limited to cities or to major hospitals. In 1951, a doctor working in a rural hospital in DRC reported transfusing blood to treat anemia from malaria in more than 5,000 infants beginning in 1943. He collected fresh blood for each transfusion from a parent, relative, or member of the clinic staff. For children with mild anemia, he reported intramuscular injections of blood. He recommended that 'all dispensaries, even small ones, should be able to manage ordinary blood transfusions' and that 'medical assistants...can be trained to transfuse infants' and can do so 'in the bush in an emergency and with minimum material support...'[37]

Because blood banks were not well-developed – due in part to lack of or unreliable refrigeration – doctors often transfused fresh blood after simple tests to match blood type. Most blood was collected from replacement or paid donors. Relying on replacement donors 'could rapidly degenerate into a system of unofficially paid donors, recruited on behalf of the relatives by "Captain Blood" operating in the local lorry-park.'[38] Repeat donors could transmit bloodborne pathogens to other donors if needles and tubes used to withdraw blood were reused without sterilization. In this way, one HIV-infected donor could infect not only the patients to whom he or she donated (sold) blood, but also other donors and, indirectly, other patients.

When HIV testing started in the 1980s, blood donors in Central Africa were often found to have higher HIV prevalence than adults in the general population. Very likely this was the situation in the 1970s as well. From their history of transfusions in Africa, Schneider and

Drucker conclude that 'transfusions may have played a significant role in the origins of the disease.'[39]

Collecting blood plasma

For donors, selling plasma – blood with the cells removed – is more dangerous than selling blood. The procedures to separate plasma from cells and to re-inject the cells provide opportunities to transmit HIV from donor to donor. Moreover, people can sell plasma more often than blood. Careless procedures to collect plasma have infected donors in many countries (see Chapters 5 and 9).

From the 1960s, US and European companies that produce blood products (such as albumin, gamma globulin, and factor VIII to stop bleeding in hemophiliacs) imported plasma from developing countries.[40] During the 1970s, Kinshasa was 'one of the main centres' extracting and exporting plasma.[41] Other African countries and Haiti also exported plasma. Wherever HIV was circulating, plasma collection could have spread HIV among donors. Unfortunately, no one has looked for HIV infections among 1970s plasma donors in countries with early HIV epidemics.

(Almost all HIV infections in Europe and the US belong to the HIV-1 B clade, and can be traced to a parent virus which left Africa around 1966. No one has identified any link between plasma exports from Africa in the 1970s and early HIV epidemics in Europe and the US. Because plasma from Africa was a recognized risk to transmit hepatitis B, processors may have used African plasma for products for which processing killed the hepatitis B virus – and also the unknown HIV.)

Recognizing bloodborne pathogens: Hepatitis B virus

By mid-century, doctors recognized that liver cancer was unusually common among Africans. In 1958, a liver specialist speculated that infections that cause hepatitis might be important contributors to liver cancer and cirrhosis in Africa.[42] Because scientists had not yet identified the viruses that cause most hepatitis, this was a guess.

In 1963, Blumberg and Alter discovered an antigen (a protein that stimulates the body to produce antibodies) in the blood of someone who had received multiple transfusions. By 1966, Blumberg and colleagues showed that what they had discovered was part of the virus that caused jaundice after blood exposures.[43] The antigen they discovered is currently known as the hepatitis B virus surface antigen, which is part of the hepatitis B virus. People with the antigen have the virus. All over the world, hepatitis B was found to be a major cause of liver cancer. Blumberg received a Nobel Prize for discovering the virus.

From the late 1960s, scientists used tests for the hepatitis B virus surface antigen to measure the percentages of people infected in different communities, and to investigate risks. In the US, Europe, and Australia, infections were rare in the general population – only between 1-3 in 1,000 were infected. In rich countries, hepatitis B was, as expected, linked to recognized blood exposures, including IDU and needlestick accidents among healthcare workers.[44]

By 1970, researchers had also found that 'in many tropical areas' 3-20 percent of people carried the hepatitis B virus surface antigen.[45] This surprising finding required not only urgent changes in medical practice, but also research to explain how it could be so. Unfortunately, at this point, medical practice and medical research in Africa both took a wrong turn.

Wrong turn in medical practice

New information that large percentages of African patients carried the hepatitis B virus meant that unsterile medical procedures were a threat to transmit hepatitis B from patient to patient. Despite this new information, ministries of health and organizations providing health aid did not revise their activities to ensure use of sterile instruments, but rather extended programs with invasive procedures that were widely known to be unsafe.

In 1978, Zuckerman, at the WHO Collaborating Centre for Reference and Research on Viral Hepatitis at the London School of Hygiene and Tropical Medicine criticized careless injection practices:[46]

> ...in some parts of Africa and Asia as many as 20 percent of the population may be carriers [of the hepatitis B virus]. The risk of transmitting hepatitis by the multidose-syringe technique [i.e., filling a syringe with multiple doses, then changing needles between patients] is therefore considerable and it is imperative that an adequately sterilized or a disposable syringe and needle should be used for each individual patient.

41

Laird, who had demonstrated in the 1940s that using sterile syringes and needles prevented jaundice after syphilis treatments, seconded the warning.[47] These warnings had no apparent impact on public health programs in Africa.

Wrong turn in research

Calculating that tens of millions of residents of tropical countries were infected with the hepatitis B virus, Blumberg and co-authors opined in 1970 that 'Very few of these would have received blood transfusions or needle injections.'[48] This ignored what was generally recognized among public health experts and doctors in Africa and other tropical regions: that injections were common. Instead, hepatitis experts speculated that some populations were genetically susceptible to infection, and that the virus might transmit through mosquitoes or other insects, poor sanitation, etc.[49] Such speculations guided decades of often fruitless research.

Early research in Africa found high prevalence of hepatitis B infection among children. In a 1972 study in Senegal, for example, 12 percent of children aged less than 1 year had active infections, increasing to 16 percent by age 7-8 years.[50] Because a large proportion of children who are infected with hepatitis B in their first five years of life develop chronic, lifetime infections, high prevalence of infection among children largely explained the observed high percentages of African adults with active infections. In contrast, almost all adults who contract a hepatitis B infection are able to defeat the virus within months, and are left only with antibodies and lifetime immunity. But why were so many African children infected with hepatitis B?

Ignoring blood exposures in healthcare, research on risks for hepatitis B in African children found no answers. Mother-to-child transmission explained only a small minority of infections. For example, in a study reported in 1973, in Kenyan families with one or more children infected with hepatitis B, only 2 of 49 mothers were infected.[51] Researchers in Cote d'Ivoire found evidence of hepatitis B virus in blood from mosquitoes, but whether mosquitoes spread the virus was another matter.[52] More informative research in Papua New Guinea published in 1972 showed that presence or absence of mosquitoes in a community had no impact on prevalence of hepatitis B infection.[53]

Some studies reported suggestive evidence pointing to healthcare risks. A 1973 paper from Kenya reported a near absence of hepatitis B infection among children aged less than 2 years in a community where 'childhood immunization is not routinely available.'[54] A study in Ibadan, Nigeria, in 1974 found that hepatitis B infection was associated with injections and frequent blood tests among adults living in the inner city, but not among residents of the wealthier suburbs.[55] But no one followed the clues.

After discovering the hepatitis B virus, scientists soon developed tests for prior infection – for antibodies to hepatitis B that persist in the blood after people have defeated the virus. With these tests, studies during the 1970s and later found that 70-95 percent of African adults had past or current infections, of which 8-20 percent had current infections.

Failure on the part of public health managers in Africa to stop practices that transmitted hepatitis B was linked to parallel failure by researchers to investigate whether healthcare procedures transmitted the virus. Did researchers not look because they were influenced by public health managers who did not want to change their practices? Or did researchers on their own avoid obvious questions?

Recognizing bloodborne pathogens: Ebola

In 1976, the first two recognized outbreaks of a frightening new disease, Ebola hemorrhagic fever, made world news. The first began in southern Sudan in August and continued into November. The largest part of the outbreak centered on a hospital in Maridi. A member of the WHO team that investigated the outbreak described the hospital as an 'epidemic amplifier.'[56] Contaminated injection equipment may have infected some patients. Hospital staff who nursed patients contracted the virus. (Research during a later Ebola outbreak found virus in blood, saliva, feces, and several other bodily fluids, but not urine.)[57] People who stayed home with Ebola passed the disease to family care-givers, but not so often that this could sustain the epidemic. The disease was deadly and fast: 150 of 299 recognized cases died.[58] Characteristically, case patients fell ill a week after exposure, and died a week later.

The first recognized death in the second outbreak occurred in Yambuku, a town in north-central DRC, on 5 September 1976. The amplifier of this outbreak was a Catholic mission hospital. Every morning, the hospital allocated five syringes and needles to the nursing staff, which they reused without sterilization throughout the day to inject outpatients and inpatients. The hospital had 120 beds and an average of 200-400 outpatients per day.

Injections accounted for most of the transmissions in the first several weeks of the Yambuku outbreak. At the same time, the virus attacked nurses caring for inpatients. The hospital closed on 30 September after most of its staff fell sick. According to WHO's International Commission that investigated the outbreak, closing the hospital was 'likely...the single event of greatest importance in the eventual termination of the outbreak.'[59] Transmission occurred less frequently during home-based care, and the last death was recorded on 5 November. From September to November 1976, this outbreak killed 211 out of 237 recognized cases.[60] The Commission noted: 'All ages and both sexes were affected, but women 15-29 years of age had the highest incidence of disease, a phenomenon strongly related to attendance at prenatal and outpatient clinics at the hospital where they received injections.'[61]

During the Yambuku outbreak, 'no person whose contact was exclusively parenteral [skin-piercing] injection survived the disease.' The Commission recommended 'a national campaign to inform health personnel of the proper methods for sterilizing syringes and needles,' more reliance on oral medication, and controls on 'the activities of itinerant nurses who treat all diseases by injection.'[62]

In 1979, Ebola re-emerged in southern Sudan. As in 1976, a hospital amplified the outbreak. As before, 'The staff do not routinely practice barrier nursing and often do not sterilize needles, syringes, or other instruments used on the wards.'[63] Most infections occurred in family members of people with hospital-acquired infections. Twenty-two of 34 cases died.

HIV-2 epidemic in Guinea-Bissau linked to blood exposures

During the decades before 1981, small numbers of people across West Africa lived with HIV-2 infections. Guinea-Bissau likely had the highest HIV-2 prevalence. Tests of stored blood collected from rural communities in Guinea-Bissau during a 1980 yellow fever survey found that 11 (0.9 percent) of 1,245 children and adults were infected.[64] From Guinea-Bissau, HIV-2 reached Portugal as well as Angola and Mozambique, which were Portuguese colonies until 1975.

A study reported in Chapter 2 linked HIV-2 infections in persons born before 1955 in Guinea-Bissau to three blood exposures (injections to treat sleeping sickness and tuberculosis, and female circumcision).[65] Two studies published in 2006 link HIV-2 infections in adults born before 1973 with other – and more recent – blood exposures. Both studies found that HIV-2 infection was more common in people with scars from smallpox vaccination than in people who had not been vaccinated (smallpox vaccination was discontinued in 1980).[66] Healthcare workers remembered that 'hygiene was not always optimal in the smallpox vaccination campaigns.' The study team concluded: 'These campaigns could have contributed to the transmission of blood-born [sic] infections like HIV-2.'[67] Moreover, in one of these studies, people with scars from BCG vaccination – which has continued – were more than twice as likely to be HIV-2-positive as people without such scars.

A review of patients treated for HIV-2 in a Portuguese hospital during 1997-2002 (most of whom were from former Portuguese colonies Guinea-Bissau and Cape Verde) reported that the concentration of infections in older age groups was[68]

> not compatible with predominant sexual transmission, which would result in a more even distribution through all age groups. These facts point to parenteral exposure (increased use of injections, vaccination campaigns, blood and its derivatives, nosocomial infection, and some traditional practices) as the principle route for the spread of this virus during the epidemic period.

Thus, findings from multiple recent studies support the view that many if not most HIV-2 infections have been from blood exposures.

HIV-1 spreads out of Africa

During the 1970s, probably the fastest growing HIV epidemics in the world concentrated in IDUs and MSMs in major cities in North America. What was required to ignite these epidemics was that HIV reach an IDU who shared injection equipment or an MSM with multiple sex partners. Once HIV began to circulate among either of these groups, it would reach the other, because many MSMs were also IDUs. [69]

More than a half dozen instances have been documented in which people contracted HIV infections in Africa and returned to Europe or North America before 1981.[70] Infected returnees include the Norwegian sailor already mentioned, a pilot transfused in Kisangani in 1976, and a Belgian living in DRC, who retired to Belgium in 1968. All of these known infections, and no doubt many others that are unknown, did not reach IDUs or MSMs, and died out without igniting or contributing to HIV epidemics.

Analyses of HIV sequences provide information about the chain of infection that led from Africa to North American and European IDUs and MSMs. Most HIV in North America, Europe, and Haiti belongs to the HIV-1 B clade. From sequences of B clade HIV collected in North America, two estimated dates for the last common ancestor are 1968 and 1969.[71] Including HIV from Haiti, the estimated date recedes to 1966. These analyses present strong evidence that B clade HIV-1 began to spread within Haiti around 1966, and reached North America from Haiti around 1969.

After the chaotic end of Belgian rule in DRC in 1960, UNESCO arranged for educated French-speaking Haitians to work in DRC.[72] If HIV could infect Europeans and North Americans in Africa before 1981 – as it did – it could certainly infect Haitians. This could have occurred through blood or sexual exposures. Similarly, the multiplication of HIV infections in Haiti, as in Africa, occurred through an unknown mix of blood and sexual exposures.

Many people have speculated that HIV passed from Haiti to North America and Europe through MSMs visiting Haiti for low-cost commercial sex. However, if HIV reached North America in the late 1960s, this probably did not occur through MSM sex tourism to Haiti, which did not develop until the 1970s. In the late 1960s, an alternate scenario for the beginning of North America's HIV epidemic is that a Haitian immigrant IDU shared syringes and needles with other IDUs in Miami, New York, or elsewhere. Supporting this scenario, there is some evidence that HIV had already infected substantial numbers of IDUs in the US as early as 1971-72.[73] Another possibility is that plasma imported from Haiti (before Haiti blocked plasma exports in the early

1970s)[74] might have gone into blood products that infected an MSM or IDU.

Testing of stored blood samples collected from MSMs in San Francisco reveal 4.9 percent to be HIV-positive in 1978, increasing to 13.5 percent in 1979.[75] This observed rate of epidemic expansion – doubling in 8 months – roughly agrees with an estimated date of 1969 for the introduction of B clade HIV to the US. If, for example, the number of B clade infections in North America and Europe doubled every 8 months, starting from one infection in 1969, there would have been 1,000 in 1975, and 250,000 in 1981 – which is not far from the estimated number of infections in North America and Europe at that time.

With this scenario one could expect several hundred AIDS cases in North America and Europe before 1981. The US Centers for Disease Control and Prevention (CDC) – looking back from 1981 and later – identified 100 AIDS cases in the US before 1981.[76] The earliest well-established AIDS case in North America, Europe, and Haiti that is not directly linked to Africa was reported in a bisexual musician from Cologne, Germany, whose symptoms began in 1976.[77] Many cases may have been missed. For example, early AIDS cases among IDUs may have been diagnosed as tuberculosis or otherwise overlooked.

From the US and Europe, the B clade spread not later than the early 1980s to Australia, Japan, South Africa, South Korea, Thailand and elsewhere through IDUs, MSMs, and blood products (especially factor VIII for hemophiliacs).

Unsterile healthcare, unresolved questions

Healthcare procedures contributed to HIV transmission in Africa and Haiti during this period. Recent research has been able to identify blood exposures before 1980 as risks for HIV-2 infection. Healthcare procedures that spread HIV-2 would have been even more likely to spread HIV-1. But was healthcare a major or minor factor in HIV-1's epidemic expansion? New information from sequencing, from stored blood, and from other sources can be expected, over time, to fill in more of the picture of the HIV epidemic during this period.

[1] Low-Beer D. 'The distribution of early acquired immune deficiency syndrome cases and conditions for the establishment of new epidemics', *Phil Trans R Soc Lond B*, 2001, 356: 927-31.

[2] Desmyter J, Goubau P, Chamaret S, et al. 'Anti-LAV/HTLV-III in Kinshasa mothers in 1970 and 1980 [abstract]', *2nd Int Conf AIDS*, Paris, 23-25 June 1986, abstract s17g.

[3] Nzilambi N, De Cock KM, Forthal DN, et al. 'The prevalence of infection with human immunodeficiency virus over a 10-year period in rural Zaire', *N Eng J Med*, 1988, 318: 276-9.

[4] Morvan J, Carteron B, Laroche R, et al. 'Enquete sero-epidemiologique sur les infections a HIV au Burundi entre 1980 et 1981', *Bull Soc Pathol Exot*, 1989, 82: 130-40.

[5] Sonnet J, Michaux J-L, Zech F, et al. 'Early AIDS cases originating from Zaire and Burundi (1962-1976)', *Scand J Infect Dis*, 1987, 19: 511-7; Vangroenweghe D. 'The earliest cases of human immunodeficiency virus type 1 group M in Congo-Kinshasa, Rwanda and Burundi and the origin of acquired immune deficiency syndrome', *Phil Trans Roy Soc Land B*, 2001, 356: 923-5.

[6] Molez J-F. 'The historical question of acquired immunodeficiency syndrome in the 1960s in the Congo River basin area in relation to cryptococcal meningitis', *Am J Trop Med Hyg*, 1998, 58: 273-6.

[7] Giraldo G, Beth E, Kyalwazi SK. 'Role of cytomegalovirus in Kaposi's sarcoma', in: Williams AO, O'Conor GT, De-The GB, et al. (eds), *Virus-Associated Cancers in Africa*. Oxford: Oxford University Press, 1984. pp. 583-606.

[8] Hooper E. *The River*. London: Penguin, 2000. pp. 762-7.

[9] Cook PJ, Burkitt DP. 'Cancer in Africa', *Br Med Bull*, 1971, 27: 14-20. p. 19.

[10] Hooper E. *The River*.

[11] US Census (US) Bureau. *HIV/AIDS Surveillance Data Base, June 2003 Release*. Washington, DC: US Census Bureau, 2003.

[12] Rambaut A, Robertson DL, Pybus OG, et al. 'Phylogeny and the origin of HIV-1', *Nature*, 2001, 410: 1047-8; Archer J, Robertson DL, 'Understanding the diversification of HIV-1 groups M and O', *AIDS*, 2007, 21: 1693-700.

[13] Vidal N, Mulanga C, Bazepeo SE, et al. 'Distribution of HIV-1 variants in the Democratic Republic of Congo suggests increase in subtype C in Kinshasa between 1997 and 2002', *J Acquir Immune Defic Syndr*, 2005, 40: 456-62.

[14] Travers SAA, Clewley JP, Glynn JR, et al. 'Timing and reconstruction of the most recent common ancestor of the subtype C clade of human immunodeficiency virus type 1', *J Virol*, 2004, 78: 10501-6.

[15] Vidal N, Niyongabo T, Nduwimana J, et al. 'HIV type 1 diversity and antiretroviral drug resistance mutations in Burundi', *AIDS Res Hum Retroviruses*, 2007, 23: 175-80.

[16] Los Alamos National Laboratory. *HIV Sequence Database*. Available at: http://www.hiv.lanl.gov/content/hiv-db (accessed 26 August 2007).

[17] Chin J. *The AIDS Pandemic*. Abingdon, UK: Radcliffe Publishing, 2007. p. 37.

[18] World Bank. *African Development Indicators 1998/99*. Washington DC: World Bank, 1998.

[19] Carael M. 'Sexual behavior', in: Cleland D, Ferry B (eds), *Sexual Behavior and AIDS in the Developing World*. London: Taylor and Francis, 1995. pp. 75-123.

[20] Merlin M, Josse R, Trebucq A, et al. 'Surveillance epidemologique du syndrome d'immunodepression acquise dans six etats d'Afrique centrale', *Med Trop*, 1988, 48: 381-9.

[21] Auvert B, Buve A, Ferry B, et al. 'Ecological and individual level analysis of risk factors for HIV infection in four urban populations in sub-Saharan Africa with different levels of HIV infection', *AIDS*, 2001, 15 (suppl 4): S15-30.

[22] Cattand P. 'L'epidemiologie de la trypanosomiase humaine Africaine: une histoire multifactorielle complexe', *Med Trop*, 2001, 61: 313-22.

[23] Guthe T. 'Clinical, serological and epidemiological features of *Framboesia tropica* (yaws) and its control in rural communities', *Acta Derm Venereol*, 1969, 49: 343-68.

[24] Fenner F, Henderson DA, Arita I, et al. *Smallpox and its Eradication*. Geneva: WHO, 1988. p. 574.

[25] Ibid., pp. 967-8.

[26] Ibid., p. 935.

[27] Gordon H. 'Syringe-transmitted hepatitis [letter]', *Brit Med J*, 1978, 2: 953.

[28] Van Lerberghe W, de Bethune X, De Brouwere V. 'Hospitals in sub-Saharan Africa: Why we need more of what does not work as it should', *Trop Med Int Health*, 1997, 2: 799-808.

[29] Declaration of Alma-Ata International Conference on Primary Health Care, Alma-Ata 6-12 September 1978. Available at:
http://www.who.int/hpr/NPH/docs/declaration_almaata.pdf (accessed 26 August 2007).

[30] Van der Geest S. 'The illegal distribution of Western medicines in developing countries: pharmacists, drug peddlers, injection doctors and others. A bibliographic exploration', *Med Anthrop*, 1982, 6: 197-219.

[31] Wyatt HV. 'The popularity of injections in the third world: Origins and consequences for poliomyelitis', *Soc Sci Med*, 1984, 19: 911-15.

[32] Beheyt P. 'Contribution a l'etude des hepatites en Afrique: L'hepatite epidemique et l'hepatite par inoculation', *Ann Soc Belge Med Trop*, 1953, 33: 297-338. p. 335. Gisselquist translated the quote.

[33] Guyer B, Candy D. 'Injectable antimalarial therapy in tropical Africa: Iatrogenic disease and wasted medical resources', *Trans R Soc Trop Med Hygiene*, 1979, 73: 230-2.

[34] Drucker E, Alcabes PG, Marx PA. 'The injection century: massive unsterile injections and the emergence of human pathogens', *Lancet*, 2001, 358: 1989-92.

[35] Schneider WH, Drucker E. 'Blood transfusions in the early years of AIDS in sub-Saharan Africa', *Am J Pub Health*, 2006, 96: 984-94.

[36] Ibid.

[37] Pieters G. 'Service de transfusion sanguine pour nourrissons congolais en zone rurale', *Ann Soc Belge Med Trop*, 1951, 31: 661-81. pp. 679-80. Gisselquist translated the quote.

[38] Fleming AF. 'HIV and blood transfusion in sub-Saharan Africa', *Transfus Sci*, 1997, 18: 167-79. p. 168.

[39] Schneider WH, Drucker E. 'Blood transfusions'. p. 993.

[40] WHO. 'Utilization and supply of human blood and blood products: Information provided by the Director-General', Geneva: WHO, 1975. Doc. no. A28/WP/6.

[41] Jones P. 'AIDS: The African connection? [letter]' *Br Med J*, 1985, 290: 932.

[42] Steiner PE. 'Some aspects of infectious hepatitis', *Ann Soc Belge Med Trop*, 1958, 38: 359-64.

[43] Blumberg BS, Sutnick AI, London WT, et al. 'Australia antigen and hepatitis', *N Eng J Med*, 1970, 283: 349-54.

[44] Cherubin CE, Hargrove RL, Prince AM. 'The serum hepatitis related antigen (SH) in illicit drug users', *Am J Epidemiol*, 1970, 91: 510-17; Koff RS, Isselbacher KJ. 'Changing concepts in the epidemiology of viral hepatitis', *N Eng J Med*, 1968, 278: 1371-80.

[45] Blumberg BS et al. 'Australia antigen and hepatitis'. p. 353.

[46] Zuckerman AJ. 'Syringe-transmitted hepatitis [letter]', *Brit Med J*, 1978, 2: 696.

[47] Laird SM. 'Syringe-transmitted hepatitis [letter]', *Brit Med J*, 1978, 2: 953.

[48] Blumberg BS et al. 'Australia antigen and hepatitis'. p. 351.

[49] Prince AM. 'Prevalence of serum-hepatitis-related antigen (SH) in different geographic regions', *Am J Trop Med Hyg*, 1970, 19: 872-9; Szmuness W, Prince AM, Diebolt G, et al. 'The epidemiology of hepatitis B infections in Africa: Results of a pilot survey in the Republic of Senegal', *Am J Epidemiol*, 1973, 98: 104-10.

[50] Ibid.

[51] Bagshawe A, Nganda TN. 'Hepatitis B antigen in a rural community in Kenya', *Trans R Soc Trop Med Hyg*, 1973, 67: 663-70.

[52] Brotman B, Prince AM, Godfrey HR, 'Role of arthropods in transmission of hepatitis-B virus in the tropics', *Lancet*, 1973; i: 1305-8.

[53] Hawkes RA, Vale TG, Marshall ID, et al. 'Contrasting seroepidemiology of Australia antigen and arbovirus antibodies in New Guinea', *Am J Epidemiol*, 1972, 95: 228-37.

[54] Bagshawe A, Nganda TN. 'Hepatitis B antigen'. p. 668.

[55] Olumide EA. 'The distribution of hepatitis B surface antigen in Africa and the tropics: Report of a population study in Nigeria', *Int J Epidemiol*, 1976; 5: 279-89.

[56] Garrett L. *The Coming Plague*. New York: Penguin, 1995. p. 148.

[57] Bausch DG, Towner JS, Dowell SF, et al. 'Assessment of the risk of Ebola virus transmission from bodily fluids and fomites', *J Infect Dis*, 2007, 196 (suppl 2): S142-7.

[58] 'Viral haemorrhagic fever', *Wkly Epidemiol Rec*, 1977, 52: 177-80.

[59] International Commission. 'Ebola haemorrhagic fever in Zaire, 1976', *Bull WHO*, 1978, 56: 271-93. p. 280.

[60] 'Viral haemorrhagic fever'.

[61] International Commission. 'Ebola haemorrhagic fever in Zaire, 1976'.

[62] Ibid. pp. 280, 290.

[63] Baron RC, McCormick JB, Zubeir OA. 'Ebola virus disease in southern Sudan: Hospital dissemination and intrafamilial spread', *Bull WHO*, 1983, 61: 997-1003. p. 997.

[64] Piedade J, Venenno T, Prieto E, et al. 'Longstanding presence of HIV-2 infection in Guinea-Bissau (West Africa)', *Acta Trop*, 2000, 76: 119-24.

[65] Pepin J, Plamondon M, Alves AC, et al. 'Parenteral transmission during excision and treatment of tuberculosis and trypanosomiasis may be responsible for the HIV-2 epidemic in Guinea-Bissau', *AIDS*, 2006, 20: 1303-11.

[66] Jensen ML, Dave S, Schim van der Loeff M, et al. 'Vaccinia scars associated with improved survival among adults in rural Guinea-Bissau', *PLoS ONE*, 2006, 1: e101; Aaby P, Gustafson P, Roth A, et al. 'Vaccinia scars associated with better survival for adults: An observational study from Guinea-Bissau', *Vaccine*, 2006, 24: 5718-25.

[67] Ibid. p. 5722.

[68] Gomes P, Abecasis A, Almeida M, et al. 'Transmission of HIV-2', *Lancet Infect Dis*, 2003, 3: 534-6. p. 535.

[69] CDC. 'Update: acquired immunodeficiency syndrome – United States,' *MMWR*, 1986, 35: 757-66.

[70] Sonnet J et al. 'Early AIDS cases'; Hooper E. *The River*.

[71] Robbins KE, Lemey P, Pybus OG, et al. 'U.S. human immunodeficiency virus type 1 epidemic: Date of origin, population history, and characterization of early strains', *J Virol*, 2003, 77: 6359-66; Gilbert MTP, Rambaut A, Wlasiuk G, et al. 'The emergence of HIV/AIDS in the Americas and beyond', *Proc Nat Acad Sci USA*, 2007, 104: 18566-70.

[72] Vangroenweghe D. 'The earliest cases'; Molez J-F. 'The historical question'.

[73] Moore JD, Cone EJ, Alexander Jr SS. 'HTLV-III seropositivity in 1971-1972 parenteral drug abusers – A case of false positives or evidence of viral exposure? [letter]', *N Eng J Med*, 1986, 314: 1387-8.

[74] Starr D. *Blood: An epic history of medicine and commerce*, New York: HarperCollins, 2000.

[75] Foley B, Pan H, Buchbinder S, et al. 'Apparent founder effect during the early years of the San Francisco HIV type 1 epidemic (1978-1979)', *AIDS Res Hum Retroviruses*, 2000, 16: 1463-9.

[76] CDC. *HIV/AIDS Surveillance Report*, 2001, 13(1).

[77] Sterry W, Marmor M, Konrads A, et al. 'Kaposi's sarcoma, aplastic pancytopenia, and multiple infections in a homosexual (Cologne 1976) [letter]', *Lancet*, 1983; i: 924-5.

Chapter 4

RECOGNIZING AIDS IN TWO EPIDEMIC PATTERNS, 1981-84

In June 1981, doctors in Los Angeles reported five men with a rare type of pneumonia caused by a common bacterium that is seldom dangerous, because it is so easily defeated by our immune system.[1] Their pneumonia was linked to an unexplained weakness in their bodies' immune defenses. All five men were MSMs, and one was also an IDU. One month later, in July 1981, doctors in New York and California reported 30 more MSMs with unusual infections, including Kaposi's sarcoma, bacterial pneumonia, severe and persistent herpes sores, and several fungal infections.[2]

Before 1981, very likely thousands of people in Africa and scores in Europe, the US, and Haiti had already died from AIDS. Some of those cases had been recognized as unusual, but then set aside as singular and unexplained events. Clusters of cases among MSMs finally called attention to the disease.

Suspecting a new virus that spreads like the hepatitis B virus

In response to these reports, the US Centers for Disease Control and Prevention (CDC) established the Kaposi's Sarcoma and Opportunistic Infections Task Force to monitor the explosion of unusual cases and to figure out what was happening. In July 1981, CDC advised doctors to 'be alert for Kaposi's sarcoma, PC [*Pneumocystis carinii*] pneumonia, and other opportunistic infections associated with immunosuppression in homosexual men.'[3]

Early guesses about the cause of immune system defects in MSMs included an inhaled drug (amyl nitrates) that enhanced orgasms, and cytomegalovirus, a common and normally inoffensive virus. Those were some of the less threatening ideas. The scary option, recognized almost immediately,[4] was that the immune defects might be due to a previously unknown virus that had begun to circulate among MSMs, and which might transmit among others as well.

In December 1981, doctors in the US reported similar symptoms – rare infections and immune defects – in IDUs.[5] Seven months later, in

July 1982, CDC reported similar symptoms in three hemophiliacs who had injected factor VIII to stop bleeding.[6] From the mid-1970s treatment for hemophilia had progressively shifted to a more concentrated, freeze-dried form of factor VIII produced from plasma pooled from thousands of donors – a process which also pooled contaminating viruses. To preserve factor VIII activity, the product was not treated to kill viruses. The introduction of factor VIII from pooled plasma put hemophiliacs in the front lines to identify new bloodborne viruses that might enter the population.

According to Curran, who led CDC's task force on Kaposi's Sarcoma and Opportunistic Infections,[7]

> The lack of consensus regarding the cause continued until July 1982...The sudden occurrence of a new syndrome that affected primarily these three distinct populations [MSMs, IDUs, and hemophiliacs] who shared only their susceptibility to hepatitis B, convinced many investigators that a transmissible agent was the primary factor responsible for the immunologic defects characteristic of AIDS.

In mid-1982, CDC scientists named the new disease acquired immune deficiency syndrome (AIDS).

The view that AIDS was caused by a bloodborne virus – like the hepatitis B virus – gained further support in December 1982 when CDC reported AIDS in an infant 20 months old who had received blood from a man who later developed AIDS.[8] The parallel with hepatitis B was ominous. If the suspected infectious agent that caused AIDS passed from person to person like the hepatitis B virus, then MSMs and IDUs in rich countries represented only a small portion of the world's population that was at risk for AIDS.

Recognizing AIDS in Haiti and Africa

In late 1981, doctors in Miami and New York alerted CDC to Haitians with symptoms similar to what doctors were finding in MSMs.[9] In early 1982, doctors in Haiti reported 11 men with aggressive Kaposi's sarcoma, noting later that 'Drugs and homosexuality have no importance' in Haitian cases.[10] In July 1982, CDC reported AIDS in 34 Haitians in the US, including 4 women and 30 men.[11] None of the 30 men reported sex with men, and only one acknowledged IDU risks. Another early report on AIDS in Haitians noted,[12]

> An interesting common epidemiologic feature linking the Haitians, homosexuals, intravenous-drug abusers, and hemophiliacs is a high incidence of hepatitis B viral markers [i.e., hepatitis B antigens or antibodies in their blood]. About 86 per cent of Haitians reportedly have one or more serologic markers of hepatitis B infection…

In late 1981, doctors in Belgium and France began to realize that they had already seen AIDS in patients from Africa.[13] According to Jacques Leibowitch, a prominent French doctor, 'From January 1982, French experience with AIDS included Africa as one of the foci of the disease.'[14] Through the end of 1984, doctors in Europe – primarily in France and Belgium – diagnosed AIDS in 111 Africans.[15] Most cases came from DRC (74 cases), Congo (12 cases), and adjacent countries in Central and East Africa, including Cameroon, Gabon, CAR, Chad, Burundi, Rwanda, Uganda, and Zambia (1-3 cases each). A 1984 report on 23 Africans – 14 men and 9 women – diagnosed with AIDS or AIDS-related symptoms in Belgium noted that most had evidence of past or current infection with hepatitis B. The authors reasoned that 'Since the distribution of AIDS seems to be parallel with that of hepatitis B viral infection, one may expect an extension of the syndrome in Central Africa.'[16]

In October 1983, the US National Institute for Health sent a team of US and European scientists to Kinshasa, DRC, to look for AIDS cases. In three weeks, the team identified 38 patients (20 men and 18 women) with AIDS in four hospitals. Diagnoses were based on symptoms and on tests showing immune system defects. No patients reported MSM or IDU risks. The study team found that injections were common, and were 'often given with unsterilized needles or syringes.' Even so, the team reported a 'strong indication of heterosexual transmission.'[17]

Also in October 1983, another team of European scientists funded by the Belgian government asked doctors at Rwanda's premier hospital, the Centre Hospitalier de Kigali, to identify AIDS cases. This approach identified 26 patients – 17 men, 7 women, and 2 children – with AIDS. Noting that 11 of 17 men with AIDS frequented prostitutes, and that 3 of 7 women were prostitutes, the team speculated that 'heterosexual promiscuity, and contact with prostitutes could be risk factors for African AIDS.' The team also noted that 'Poor hygiene during medical procedures might also play an important role in the transmission of a blood-borne agent.'[18]

Two epidemic patterns

Early views of the AIDS epidemic suffered from understandable confusions. Initially, public health officials did not realize the full range of symptoms associated with AIDS. The reported sudden upsurge of AIDS cases in the US, Europe, Haiti, and Africa around 1980 is almost certainly due in part to a lot of unrecognized and unreported cases in the 1970s. Doctors may have forgotten AIDS-related symptoms in patients seen before 1981. Even when doctors remembered, they may have been loath to associate their clinics or their patients who had died with AIDS to a stigmatized high risk group.

Not being able to test for the infection made it hard to measure the spread of the epidemic. From people who had donated or received blood and then gone on to develop AIDS or pre-AIDS symptoms, scientists could see that people were infected for some time before they developed symptoms. But without knowing the length of the latency period (the time from infection to symptoms) it was difficult to estimate how many were infected. If AIDS cases were the tip of the iceberg, a longer latency period meant there was a bigger, hidden iceberg. One study in 1984 estimated an average latency period of 10.5 months.[19] This was far from the true period, which is closer to 10 years. Also, because of the latency period, it was not possible from the absence of AIDS cases in a city or population to say the epidemic had not already reached there.

Even so, by observing the distribution of AIDS cases, public health experts were able to trace the spread of the infectious agent across countries and to determine some of the important risks. Through December 1984, 33 countries – 15 in the Americas, 17 in Europe, and Australia – reported a cumulative total of almost 10,000 AIDS cases to the WHO.[20] The US accounted for more than 80 percent of these cases. Although doctors had seen many Africans with AIDS, no African government reported any AIDS cases to WHO through the end of 1984.

Concentrated epidemics with identified risks

In the US through December 1984, CDC reported more than 14 men for every woman with AIDS, and 93 percent of cases were MSMs or IDUs. At the same time, CDC identified 'heterosexual contact' with 'a person with AIDS or at risk for AIDS,' such as an MSM or IDU, as the risk for 5 men and 54 women – less than 1 percent of AIDS cases.[21] Similarly, in Europe through December 1984, 92 percent of AIDS cases were MSMs, IDUs, hemophiliacs, or recipients of blood transfusions (setting aside Africans and Haitians diagnosed in Europe).[22]

Even before scientists had found the pathogen that caused AIDS, the most important risks in concentrated epidemics were pretty well understood. Whatever caused AIDS passed – like the hepatitis B virus – through anal sex among MSMs and through blood exposures when IDUs shared injection equipment.

Generalized epidemics with undetermined risks

On the other hand, AIDS in Haiti and Africa did not concentrate in MSMs and IDUs, but was found in men and women in the general population. This distribution of AIDS cases posed the question: what proportion of cases was from heterosexual exposures, and what proportion was from blood exposures?

Some experts jumped to conclusions from insufficient evidence. Piot, the leader of the team that went to Kinshasa in 1983 to look for AIDS cases, recounted his thoughts on visiting Mama Yemo Hospital: 'And then I knew what it was. I said, "Aha, this is bad news. It must be heterosexual," because there were more women than men.'[23] Similarly, Joe McCormick, who organized the team, remembered:[24]

> The major insight was – and this was the substance of a substantial discussion when I got back – the major insight was that there was an equal ratio of male to female cases. It was very clear from this that we were looking at heterosexual transmission…This was a real revelation.

Others remained unconvinced that heterosexual (penile-vaginal) transmission could account for most AIDS cases in Africa and Haiti. In November 1983, WHO organized an international meeting of experts 'to assess the present situation of AIDS' and to help countries to work together to address the epidemic. The memorandum from the meeting recognized that 'Spouses of AIDS patients have also been shown to be at an increased risk...' but was cautious in attributing AIDS to heterosexual promiscuity. 'Whether persons with multiple heterosexual sex partners are at greater risk of acquiring AIDS is unknown...' The memorandum speculated that 'injections with unsterile needles and syringes may play a role' in tropical countries.[25] One of several recommendations to prevent AIDS urged training medical staff to use only sterilized syringes and needles.

Different responses to suspected risks in blood exposures

Countries with concentrated epidemics

In November 1982, even before scientists had found the virus that caused AIDS, CDC advised medical staff to avoid needlestick accidents and to wear gloves and other protective clothing when working with suspected AIDS patients.[26] To prevent patient-to-patient transmission of whatever caused AIDS, CDC recommended existing practices to prevent patient-to-patient transmission of hepatitis B virus – which meant disinfecting equipment (generally autoclaving, or boiling under pressure) or discarding it after use. During the 1980s and later, autoclaving instruments, wearing protective gear, and other infection control practices to protect patients and healthcare workers from HIV and other pathogens have been collectively identified as 'universal precautions,' and later 'standard precautions.'

CDC, which is an agency of the US central government, did not (and does not) have the authority to require public and private healthcare providers throughout the US to follow its recommendations. CDC's recommendations had impact in the US and in other countries because they influenced ideas about what were acceptably safe practices. In some cases, other central or sub-national government agencies which funded or regulated healthcare institutions adopted CDC's recommendations into their regulations.

Healthcare providers in rich countries are subject to public and in some cases private licenses, certification, and inspections. Inspectors and regulators – along with providers – are alert to mistakes and to complaints from patients because failure to respond could lead to civil suits, criminal charges, and (for providers) loss of licenses or accreditation, and thus loss of income. Much of the 'stick' that enforces healthcare safety in rich countries is the opportunity for patients to sue whoever is careless. In addition, prosecutors for national or sub-national governments can charge regulators and inspectors as well as providers with crimes ranging from carelessness to murder if they allow or provide healthcare that does not meet accepted safety standards. On a case-by-case basis, courts – judges and juries – decide what are accepted standards. CDC's recommendations influence court decisions.

While healthcare regulators and providers in rich countries followed CDC's advice to strengthen infection control practices in response to the suspected new virus, they rejected CDC's advice to protect recipients of blood transfusions and blood products. During 1982, doctors in the US identified AIDS in one recipient of a blood transfusion and in six hemophiliacs who had received blood products. In January 1983, CDC scientists met with representatives of the US blood industry along with staff of the Food and Drug Administration (the government agency that regulates the blood industry) to discuss steps to protect recipients of blood and blood products.[27]

Because there was as yet no test for the suspected AIDS virus, CDC scientists urged organizations that collected blood and plasma to turn away donors who were at high risk for AIDS, primarily MSMs and IDUs, or to test donors not only for current hepatitis B infection, but also for prior infection (i.e., for antibodies that persist after people have defeated the virus). Antibodies showing prior hepatitis B infection were found in about 80 percent of AIDS cases and members of high-risk groups, but in only about 5 percent of other Americans. Representatives of the blood industry rejected both options, citing costs and opposing CDC's conjecture that whatever caused AIDS passed through blood. The meeting ended with no agreement.

Don Francis, who participated in the meeting as a CDC scientist, considered that failure to protect the blood supply at that time 'killed tens of thousands of hemophiliacs and transfusion recipients in the United States and around the world.' He attributed the failure to 'laziness, profit motive and this incredible inertia that some groups have to not change.' Producing clotting factor for hemophiliacs[28]

...was a commercial enterprise, and they had their collection facilities in impoverished parts of the world, collecting material they shouldn't have, and wanted to deny there was any risk... But that's understandable in a way, a nasty, evil profit motive.

...the blood banks were these...supposedly nonprofit organizations for the public good who were, from CDC's standpoint, killing people just because they didn't want to change their procedures...

In March 1983, the Food and Drug Administration called for self-deferral, recommending that members of high-risk groups not donate blood or plasma.[29] For almost two years, the US government relied on this weak recommendation to keep HIV out of blood and blood products. On 11 January 1985, as soon as tests for HIV infection were available in sufficient quantities, the Food and Drug Administration mandated testing all blood and blood products for HIV antibodies.[30] Most other rich countries started testing all blood and blood products in the last half of 1985.

Between 1983 to 1985, contaminated blood and blood products produced in the US and Europe infected thousands of patients and hemophiliacs throughout the world. Even after 1985, contaminated blood products continued to infect hemophiliacs as blood industry managers and regulators overlooked evidence for the continuing presence of HIV. During the 1990s, courts in France, Germany, Switzerland, and Japan convicted 16 blood industry managers and regulators of crimes ranging from 'endangering the safety of patients' and 'professional negligence' to poisoning, manslaughter, and murder.[31] More than 20 governments have arranged to pay compensation to people infected with HIV through blood or blood products.

Countries with generalized epidemics

At the beginning of the 1980s, public health managers and healthcare providers in Africa and Haiti had been careless for decades about minor blood exposures. Thus, the threat to the public to contract AIDS from blood exposures was not only much greater than in the US and Europe, but that threat could also not be addressed by tweaking the existing system. When scientists deduced in mid-1982 that a bloodborne pathogen caused AIDS, public health managers in Africa and Haiti did not immediately address routine lapses in infection control. This continued their pattern of non-response to evidence that reusing syringes and needles without sterilization led to jaundice (from the 1940s), to surveys showing high prevalence of hepatitis B infection in Africa (from the late 1960s), and to terrifying outbreaks of Ebola hemorrhagic fever (from 1976).

Finding HIV, developing tests

In January 1983, Luc Montagnier with a group of French scientists succeeded in isolating and growing the virus that caused AIDS in a cell culture. In February, they photographed it with an electron microscope. In May 1983, less than two years after AIDS had been recognized as a new disease, French scientists reported the discovery of what they suspected to be – and which was – the virus that caused AIDS.[32] Because they had grown their virus from an MSM with swollen lymph nodes (a common precursor to full-blown AIDS) they named it the lymphadenopathy associated virus, or LAV.

In April 1984, almost a year after the French team had published its results, Robert Gallo and a group of US scientists claimed to have discovered the virus that caused AIDS, and named it human T-lymphotropic virus type III (HTLV-III).[33] In August 1984, Jay Levy and a third group of scientists announced they had isolated a virus from AIDS patients in California and gave it a third name, AIDS-associated retrovirus (ARV).[34] Subsequently, in a compromise between French and US scientists, LAV was renamed the human immunodeficiency virus, or HIV.

Despite some initial confusion, US as well as French laboratories from late 1983 were working with the right virus. Scientists competed to develop tests to identify the presence of the virus and of antibodies to the virus. Researchers were able to test limited numbers of individuals for HIV infection from 1984. In early 1985, several companies put test kits on the market.

The availability of tests for HIV infection led to safer blood transfusions, allowed people to see who was infected, and facilitated research into the risks for AIDS. Two important first challenges were to map the spread of HIV infection in Africa, and to determine what proportion of infections in Africa and Haiti could be traced to sex, and what proportion was due to unsafe medical injections and other blood exposures.

[1] Gottleib MS, Schanker HM, Fan PT, et al. '*Pneumocystis* pneumonia – Los Angeles', *MMWR*, 1981, 30: 250-2. The bacterium that caused pneumonia was first identified as *Pneumocystis carinii*, but is now recognized as *P. jirovecii*. See: Morris A, Lundgren JD, Masur H, et al. 'Current epidemiology of *Pneumocystis* pneumonia', *Emerg Infect Dis*, 2004, 10: 1713-19.

[2] Friedman-Kien A, Laubenstein L, Marmor M, et al. 'Kaposi's sarcoma and *Pneumocystis* pneumonia among homosexual men – New York City and California', *MMWR*, 1981, 30: 305-8.

[3] Ibid. p. 307.

[4] Shilts R. *And the Band Played On*. New York: St. Martin's, 2000. p. 73.

[5] Masur H, Michelis MA, Greene JB, et al. 'An outbreak of community-acquired *Pneumocystis carinii* pneumonia: Initial manifestation of cellular immune dysfunction', *N Eng J Med*, 1981, 305: 1431-8.

[6] '*Pneumocystis carinii* pneumonia among persons with hemophilia A', *MMWR*, 1982, 31: 365-7.

[7] Curran JW. 'AIDS – Two years later', *N Eng J Med*, 1983, 309: 609-11. p. 609.

[8] Ammann A, Cowan M, Ware D, et al. 'Possible transfusion-associated acquired immune deficiency syndrome (AIDS) – California', *MMWR*, 1982, 31: 652-4.

[9] Garrett L. *The Coming Plague*. New York: Penguin, 1995. pp. 307-8.

[10] Liautaud B, Laroche C, Duvivier J, et al. 'Le sarcoma de Kaposi en Haiti: foyer meconnu ou recemment apparu?', *Ann Dermatol Venereol*, 1983, 110: 213-19. p. 213.

[11] Hensley GT, Moskowitz LB, Pitchenik AE, et al. 'Opportunistic infections and Kaposi's sarcoma among Haitians in the United States', *MMWR*, 1982, 31: 353-4, 360-1.

[12] Vieira J, Frank E, Spira TJ, et al. 'Acquired immune deficiency in Haitians: opportunistic infections in previously healthy Haitian immigrants', *N Eng J Med*, 1982, 308: 125-9. p. 128.

[13] Garrett L. *The Coming Plague*. pp. 290-291; Shilts R. *And the Band Played On*. p. 102.

[14] Leibowitch J. *Un virus etrange venu d'ailleurs*. Paris: Bernard Grasset, 1984. p. 50. Gisselquist translated the quote.

[15] Brunet JB, Ancelle RA. 'The international occurrence of the acquired immune deficiency syndrome', *Ann Internal Med*, 1985, 103: 670-4.

[16] Clumeck N, Sonnet J, Taelman H, et al. 'Acquired immunodeficiency syndrome in African patients', *N Eng J Med*, 1984, 310: 492-7. p. 496.

[17] Piot P, Quinn TC, Taelman H, et al. 'Acquired immunodeficiency syndrome in a heterosexual population in Zaire', *Lancet*, 1984, ii: 65-9. p. 68.

[18] Van de Perre P, Rouvroy D, Lepage P, et al. 'Acquired immunodeficiency syndrome in Rwanda', *Lancet*, 1984, ii: 62-5. p. 65.

[19] Auerbach DM, Darrow WW, Jaffe HW, et al. 'Cluster of cases of the acquired immune deficiency syndrome. Patients linked by sexual contact', *Am J Med*, 1984, 76: 487-92.

[20] Brunet JB, Ancelle RA. 'The international occurrence'.

[21] CDC. 'Acquired immunodeficiency syndrome (AIDS) weekly surveillance report – United States, 31 December 1984', Atlanta: CDC, no date. Available at: http://www.cdc.gov/hiv/topics/surveillance/resources/reports/past.htm (accessed 10 September 2006).

[22] Brunet JB, Ancelle RA. 'The international occurrence'.

[23] Public Broadcasting Service. 'Frontline: The age of AIDS: Interview with Peter Piot'. Posted May 2006. Available at: http://www.pbs.org/wgbh/pages/frontline/aids/interviews/piot.html (accessed 20 December 2006).

[24] Public Broadcasting Service. 'Frontline: The age of AIDS: Interview with Joe McCormick.' Posted May 2006. Available at: http://www.pbs.org/wgbh/pages/frontline/aids/interviews/mccormick.html (accessed 17 October 2007).

[25] 'Acquired immunodeficiency syndrome – An assessment of the present situation in the world: memorandum from a WHO meeting', *Bull WHO*, 1984, 62: 419-32. pp. 419, 425.

[26] CDC. 'Acquired immune deficiency syndrome (AIDS): Precautions for clinical and laboratory staff', *MMWR*, 1982, 31: 577-80.

[27] Shilts R. *And the Band Played On*. pp. 220-4.

[28] Public Broadcasting Service. 'The age of AIDS: Interview with Don Francis.' Posted May 2006. Available at: http://www.pbs.org/wgbh/pages/frontline/aids/interviews/francis.html (accessed 17 October 2007).

[29] CDC. 'Prevention of acquired immune deficiency syndrome (AIDS): Report of inter-agency recommendations', *MMWR*, 1983, 32: 101-3.

[30] CDC. 'Provisional public health service inter-agency recommendations for screening donated blood and plasma for antibody to the virus causing acquired immunodeficiency syndrome', *MMWR*, 1985, 34: 1-5.

[31] Weinberg PD, Hounshell J, Sherman LA, et al. 'Legal, financial, and public health consequences of HIV contamination of blood and blood products in the 1980s and 1990s', *Ann Intern Med*, 2002, 136: 312-19.

[32] Barre-Sinoussi F, Chermann JC, Rey F, et al. 'Isolation of a T-lymphotrophic retrovirus from a patient at risk for acquired immune deficiency syndrome (AIDS)', *Science*, 1983, 220: 868-71.

[33] Gallo RC, Salahuddin SZ, Popovic M, et al. 'Frequent detection and isolation of cytopathic retroviruses (HTLV-III) from patients with AIDS and at risk for AIDS', *Science*, 1984, 224: 500-3.

[34] Levy JA, Hoffman AD, Kramer SM, et al. 'Isolation of lymphocytopathic retroviruses from San Francisco patients with AIDS', *Science*, 1984, 225: 840-2.

Chapter 5

FROM FIRST TESTS TO A CONSENSUS ON RISKS, 1984-88

During 1984-88, researchers tested millions of people all over the world for HIV infection. Testing was sufficient to find where HIV had reached and to make ballpark estimates of the numbers infected. In Africa and in Haiti, public health experts faced the additional challenge of finding and closing the paths through which HIV transmitted among the general population.

First estimates: Pattern 1 or concentrated epidemics

In 1988, WHO described AIDS epidemics in the Americas (except parts of the Caribbean), Western Europe, Australia, and New Zealand as Pattern 1 epidemics, where 'most cases occur among homosexuals or bisexual males and intravenous drug users,' and 'the male-to-female sex ratio of infection ranges from 10:1 to 15:1.'[1] In countries with Pattern 1 or concentrated epidemics, surveys during 1984-88 sampled members of high-risk groups, such as MSMs attending a specific clinic. Then, to estimate the total number of people infected, information from these surveys was combined with estimates of the percentages of the population in high-risk groups.

Testing found more HIV infections than most people had expected. As of 1988, WHO estimated 2.3 to 2.8 million HIV infections in the Americas, Western Europe, Australia, and New Zealand.[2] This agreed with CDC's estimate of 1 million infections in the US in 1989, equivalent to 0.6 percent adult HIV prevalence.

Through December 1988, CDC attributed 89 percent of cumulative AIDS cases in the US to MSMs and IDUs, 3 percent to transfusions of blood and blood products, 3 percent to heterosexual exposures (setting aside persons born in countries with generalized epidemics), and a few percent to other and unknown risks.[3] Similar concentrations of AIDS cases in MSMs and IDUs appeared in Western Europe, Australia, and Canada.

First estimates: Pattern 2 or generalized epidemics in Africa and Haiti

In Africa and parts of the Caribbean, WHO described Pattern 2 epidemics, in which 'The male-to-female ratio of infection is approximately 1:1,' and IDU and MSM account for few infections.[4] In Africa and Haiti, most HIV infections spread across adults with no recognized unusual behaviors or risks. Small groups with high HIV prevalence, such as sex workers, accounted for small minorities of infections. Thus, it was necessary to survey the general population to determine the number of infections.

During 1985-90, governments of four African countries arranged national surveys. In some other countries, well-designed surveys targeted the general population in one or more cities or rural communities. Despite some questions about survey design (whether communities and individuals were chosen at random), and HIV tests (number of HIV-positive results that were false positives), these surveys provide good information about the numbers and distribution of HIV infections in Africa in 1988.

Other important data come from sentinel surveys of HIV prevalence among pregnant women attending selected clinics for antenatal care. Although HIV prevalence among women at urban antenatal clinics has generally been far greater than in all urban and rural adults, data from urban antenatal clinics is useful to compare HIV prevalence across countries and to track changes over time.

After 'a detailed meta-analysis of available seroprevalence data for each country in sub-Saharan Africa,' WHO estimated that as of 1988, 2.5 million people were living with HIV infection in generalized epidemics in Africa and the Caribbean.[5] At the same time, WHO estimated that HIV prevalence in the total population – including children – was 1.0 percent or more in 10 African countries, and 0.5 percent or more in two others (Table 5.1). Because African populations are heavily weighted towards younger ages (due to high rates of population growth, 45 percent of the population was aged 0-14 years in the late 1980s),[6] and because adults account for most HIV infections, this was roughly equivalent to estimating adult HIV prevalence of at least 2 percent and 1 percent in 10 and 2 countries respectively.

In 1988, the combined population of the 12 countries that WHO considered to have the worst HIV epidemics in Africa was 130 million. Using WHO's lower bound estimate for the percentage of the population infected in each country, these countries had at least 1.1 million infections. Thus, WHO's estimate of 2.5 million infections for countries with generalized epidemics assumed higher prevalence in some of these 12 countries, as well as some infections in other countries in Africa and in the Caribbean. But WHO did not publish these details.

Table 5.1: Countries with the worst HIV epidemics in 1988

Region, country	WHO's 1988 estimated HIV prevalence (%), all ages[7]	HIV prevalence (%) in adults:			
		General population surveys, 1985-90[8]		Urban women at antenatal clinics[9]	
		Urban	Rural	1985-86	1987-88
West Africa					
Cote d'Ivoire*	≥1.0	7.3	4.9	3	6.0
Guinea Bissau*	≥1.0		1.8[†]		6.0
Central Africa					
CAR	≥1.0	5.4[‡]		4.7	5.2
Congo	≥1.0	4.6			5.4
DRC	≥1.0			6	6.0
East Africa					
Burundi	≥1.0	11[§], 16[¶]	0.7	15	18
Rwanda	≥1.0	21	1.5	-	32
Tanzania	≥0.5			3.7	7.8
Uganda	≥1.0	7.7-29	0-12	11	24
Southern Africa					
Malawi	≥1.0			2	8.2
Zambia	≥1.0			5	12
Zimbabwe	≥0.5				
Caribbean					
Haiti					9

* Some data for these countries include HIV-2 infections.
† Survey in 1980
‡ Combined results from two surveys in Bangui in 1986-87
§ Survey includes children
¶ Survey in semi-urban areas
Sources: See references by column.

Central Africa

As of 1988, WHO estimated that at least 1 percent of the population (2 percent of adults) was HIV-positive in three countries in Central Africa: CAR, Congo, and DRC. In all three, median HIV prevalence among women attending antenatal clinics in urban areas was around 5-6 percent in 1987-88. Considering that most people lived in rural areas with lower HIV prevalence, WHO's estimate may have been a bit high for these countries.

There is some evidence for relatively slow epidemic expansion in DRC during the 1980s. In Kinshasa, 3 percent of mothers attending well-baby clinics were HIV-positive in 1980 (from stored blood).[10] In seven years – i.e., by 1987 – HIV prevalence in Kinshasa doubled to 6 percent among pregnant women at antenatal clinics. Near Yambuku in north central DRC, 5 (0.8 percent) of 659 rural adults and children were HIV-positive in 1976 (from tests of stored blood collected after the community's 1976 Ebola outbreak). In 1986 researchers went back to see what had happened. Two of the five people who had been HIV-positive in 1976 were alive and HIV-positive in 1986, while three had died with symptoms suggesting AIDS. At the same time, a new survey found that 3 (0.8 percent) of 388 rural adults were HIV-positive, which suggests stable HIV prevalence in the area from 1976 to 1986.[11]

In Cameroon, where the HIV-1 M group began, surveys in 11 rural and urban communities in 1985-87 found from 0 percent to 1 percent of adults to be HIV-positive. From this, the team that organized the surveys estimated adult HIV prevalence in Cameroon to be not more than 0.5 percent.[12]

West Africa

Among the 12 African countries with the worst HIV epidemics in 1988, WHO listed two in West Africa: Cote d'Ivoire and Guinea-Bissau. During the 1980s, HIV-1 expanded into West Africa, where HIV-2 had circulated at low levels in previous decades. By 1988, HIV-1 accounted for most HIV infections in Cote d'Ivoire and Burkina Faso. HIV-2 continued to be more common in Guinea-Bissau, Senegal, and Gambia.

Cote d'Ivoire appears to have had one of the fastest growing HIV epidemics in the 1980s. Surveys in randomly selected communities in February 1989 found 4.9 percent HIV prevalence in rural adults and 7.3 percent in urban adults, excluding Abidjan (see Table 5.1). These results include HIV-1 and HIV-2 infections. If these results are reliable, adult HIV prevalence in Cote d'Ivoire was around 6 percent in 1988 (two-fifths of the population was urban), and Cote d'Ivoire along with Uganda (see below) had the two worst HIV epidemics.

For Guinea-Bissau, tests of stored blood from a 1980 rural survey found 0.9 percent HIV-2 prevalence in children and adults (as reported in Chapter 3), including 1.8 percent HIV-2 prevalence in adults (9 infected of 510 tested), and there were no HIV-1 infections. Through the 1980s, HIV-1 remained rare in Guinea-Bissau. Although some studies during the 1980s reported higher HIV-2 prevalence in some communities, the persistence of higher prevalence in older people suggests that Guinea-Bissau's HIV-2 epidemic expanded little, if at all, during the 1980s.

East Africa

At the end of the 1980s, several countries east of DRC appeared to have some of the worst epidemics in Africa. As of 1987-88, median HIV prevalence in selected urban antenatal clinics ranged from 18 percent to 32 percent in Burundi, Rwanda, and Uganda. WHO estimated at least 1 percent HIV prevalence in the total population in all three countries in 1988, and at least 0.5 percent in Tanzania.

A national survey in Rwanda in 1986 found that 21 percent of adults were HIV-positive in urban areas (with 5.8 percent of the population), but only 1.5 percent in rural areas (see Table 5.1). Combining rural and urban data, estimated adult HIV prevalence across the country was 2.7 percent. This was, notably, less than one-tenth the 32 percent HIV prevalence reported from an urban antenatal clinic in Kigali in 1988!

Somewhat similar data are available for Burundi. A national survey in 1989-90 reported 11 percent HIV prevalence among adults and children in urban areas, 16 percent among adults in semi-urban areas, and 0.7 percent among adults in rural areas (see Table 5.1). The information I have from this survey does not show HIV prevalence among urban adults, or the percentage of the population that lived in semi-urban areas. But because most of the population was rural, if the survey's results are at all accurate for rural areas, Burundi's adult HIV prevalence could not have been much more than about 2 percent in 1988 – matching WHO's lower-bound estimate.

Uganda very likely had the highest HIV prevalence in 1988. The government of Uganda arranged a national survey in 1987-88. Several accounts of this survey report HIV prevalence in various regions ranging from 0 percent to 12 percent in rural adults and from 7.7

69

percent to 29 percent in urban adults (see Table 5.1). Two second-hand accounts of survey results report estimates of 600,000-800,000 infections in Uganda,[13] which would be equivalent to 7-10 percent adult HIV prevalence. Considering that HIV prevalence may have been lower in several regions not surveyed, that false positives were a problem,[14] and that only 11 percent of Uganda's population was urban, HIV prevalence may have been near or even below the low end of that range.

Kagera Region, west of Lake Victoria, had the worst HIV epidemic in Tanzania in the 1980s. Surveys of the general population in Kagera Region in 1989 found 24 percent of adults to be HIV-positive in Bukoba town, 10 percent in adjacent rural communities, 4.5 percent in more remote districts, and only 0.4 percent in the most remote districts in the Region.[15] Through 1988, HIV prevalence reached 7.8 percent among women attending an antenatal clinic in Dar es Salaam. Considering that 20 percent of Tanzania's population was urban in 1988, even though HIV had not reached much of the country, adult HIV prevalence across Tanzania may well have exceeded WHO's lower-bound estimate of 1% in 1988.

Southern Africa

WHO listed three countries in Southern Africa – Malawi, Zambia, and Zimbabwe – among the 12 African countries with the worst HIV epidemics in 1988. Through 1988, infections in Zambia, Zimbabwe, and Malawi appear to have concentrated in large cities and in Zambia's Copperbelt, adjacent to DRC. Even so, HIV prevalence in urban antenatal women in these three countries was much lower than in Rwanda and Burundi. However, the epidemic was growing fast. During 1985-87, HIV prevalence among women at urban antenatal clinics in Malawi and Zambia more than doubled to 8-12 percent (see Table 5.1; comparable data are not available from Zimbabwe).

The Caribbean

WHO provided no estimates for HIV prevalence in 1988 in Haiti and in other Caribbean countries considered to have generalized epidemics. Based on surveys among blood donors, pregnant women, and other groups in urban areas (there was little information from rural

70

areas), HIV prevalence in Haiti was comparable to what was found in DRC.[16] Similar surveys in other Caribbean countries generally found much less HIV through 1988.

First estimates: Pattern 3 HIV epidemics in the rest of the world

In 1988, WHO characterized epidemics in North Africa, the Middle East, Central and Eastern Europe, Asia, and most of the Pacific as Pattern 3 epidemics, with 'recent onset of the HIV/AIDS pandemic (mid to late 1980s),' and with few AIDS cases to date. In this vast region with most of the world's population, WHO estimated 100,000 HIV infections in 1988 – less than 1 infection in 20,000 adults. Although most countries with Pattern 3 epidemics 'have not as yet shown predominant modes of HIV transmission,'[17] some countries were already showing signs of Pattern 1 or 2 epidemics.

Information from south India through 1988 suggested the emergence of a Pattern 2 or generalized epidemic. In 1986, tests on 102 women in sex work in Tamil Nadu found 10 to be HIV-positive.[18] Very likely HIV had been circulating in India for some time when it was discovered, because expanded testing in 1987-88 in multiple sites across thousands of kilometers found infections in pregnant women, sex workers, patients with tuberculosis or sexually transmitted disease, and MSMs. Most HIV in India belongs to the HIV-1 C clade, and is related to HIV that circulates in much of Southern and East Africa. Family ties between India and Africa provided many opportunities for HIV to reach India. Analyses of HIV sequences from India might reveal the dates that several C clade viruses reached India and then multiplied to contribute to India's epidemic.

Through 1988, Thailand's HIV epidemic looked like a Pattern 1 or concentrated epidemic. The first known HIV infection in Thailand was in an MSM returning from the US with AIDS in 1984. He most likely acquired his infection in the US, and did not pass it to anyone in Thailand. A year later, in 1985, doctors in Bangkok found an HIV-positive male sex worker who had not lived outside Thailand.[19] Through 1987, doctors identified approximately 200 HIV infections. Then, in nine months from late 1987 to September 1988, HIV prevalence in IDUs attending drug treatment clinics in Bangkok soared from 1 percent to 43 percent.[20] A royal amnesty in December 1987 likely

71

contributed to this epidemic surge by releasing HIV-positive IDUs from prison into the community.

Assessing generalized epidemics: Who was infected?

Researchers looking for high-risk groups in Africa and the Caribbean found few MSMs and IDUs (except some MSMs in Haiti).[21] However, researchers found other groups that characteristically had higher HIV prevalence than other adults, including women, women in sex work, patients, urban residents, people with high socio-economic status, and blood donors.

Whereas women were much less likely than men to be HIV-positive in countries with concentrated epidemics, women in Africa were more often infected than men. For example, among thousands of patients found to be HIV-positive in Kinshasa in 1986, the ratio of women to men was 1.3 to 1.[22]

High rates of HIV infection among women in sex work are characteristic of generalized epidemics (see Table 5.2). In one of the first studies that tested African blood for HIV, Van de Perre found 88 percent of a sample of sex workers in Rwanda in 1984 to be HIV-positive.[23] As later studies showed, this was unusually high, not only for sex workers in Africa but for all high-risk groups in all countries.

During 1984-88, hundreds of studies found high HIV prevalence among various categories of patients (Table 5.2). There were many reasons for patients to be HIV-positive, so the sources of their infections were not clear. People with HIV infection and weakened immune systems are more likely to get tuberculosis, genital ulcers, diarrhea, and other conditions that bring them to clinics. On the other hand, sexually transmitted diseases may have been markers for sexual behaviors that are risks for HIV infection. In addition, people who attended clinics for long-term or repeat treatment (such as for tuberculosis) may have been infected during treatment.

Within each African country, urban adults had higher HIV prevalence than rural adults. The difference varied from country to country.

During 1985-88, many studies across Africa found that high socioeconomic status was a risk for HIV infection. Studies in Kinshasa reported higher HIV prevalence in administrators or higher-paid staff vs. other staff at a hospital,[24] bank, and textile factory.[25] Among inpatients and outpatients in Zambia in 1985, HIV prevalence increased progressively from 8 percent among those with 0-4 years of education up to 33 percent for those with more than 14 years of education.[26]

Table 5.2: HIV prevalence (percentages) in selected populations in generalized epidemics, 1984-88

Region, country	Women in sex work*	Patients at clinics treating sexually transmitted disease*	Inpatients: Median [range]†	Blood donors: Median [range]†
West Africa				
Cote d'Ivoire‡	29	7.7	34 [6.8-70]	12 [2.8-19]
Guinea-Bissau‡			14 [9.8-16]	8.5 [5.1-9.8]
Central Africa				
CAR	14	18	6.5 [1.1-9.7]	12
Congo	49	18	32 [7.7-38]	7.1 [3.4-14]
DRC	35		31 [4.1-87]	6.0 [1.0-9.0]
East Africa				
Burundi				8.8 [8.3-9.2]
Rwanda		62		18 [11-20]
Tanzania	42	25	10 [2.3-34]	5.1 [0.7-11]
Uganda		52	37 [27-38]	16 [9.2-23]
Southern Africa				
Malawi	56	62	21 [4.5-29]	20
Zambia		22	19 [15-27]	14 [6.0-19]
Zimbabwe		52	5.1	3.0 [2.3-37]
Caribbean				
Haiti	53	-	49 [35-63]	4.0 [2.2-16]

* These columns show medians from sentinel surveys in urban areas reported by WHO[27]; for each country, the columns show the last available median from 1985-88, except that for patients with sexually transmitted disease in Congo, CAR, Malawi, Uganda, and Zimbabwe, the column shows the first reported medians from 1989-90.

† These columns summarize data compiled by the US Census Bureau[28] from studies that tested at least 50 inpatients or 100 blood donors (excluding data identified by the US Census Bureau as 'data of unknown quality').

‡ Includes HIV-2 infections.

Sources: See references in notes for each column.

Although HIV screening of transfused blood was absent or erratic in most of Africa during 1985-88, many hospitals tested at least some blood intended for transfusion. HIV prevalence in blood donors often exceeded prevalence in urban adults. Many donors, including replacement donors recruited by patients' families, were paid, repeat donors.

Assessing generalized epidemics: Sexual transmission

From 1984, the CDC began to list 'heterosexual contact...with a person with AIDS or at risk for AIDS' as a high-risk category in its reports of AIDS cases in the US.[29] Studies in the US and Europe during 1984-88 found that as many as 25 percent or more of the spouses of HIV-positive IDUs, MSMs, or hemophiliacs were also infected.[30] This was on the one hand reassuring, because HIV seemed to transmit inefficiently through penile-vaginal sex. But on the other hand, it was disturbing, because it meant that people were at risk from heterosexual partners. Where HIV had invaded the general population – as in Africa and Haiti – this called for programs to warn people to be aware of risk, and to use condoms with heterosexual partners who might be HIV-positive.

However, the finding that HIV transmitted (inefficiently) through penile-vaginal sex did not by itself explain generalized HIV epidemics. If, as many people believed, most HIV-infected adults in Africa and Haiti acquired their infections from heterosexual partners, then it was necessary to explain how heterosexual sex could transmit HIV so much more extensively in Africa and Haiti than in the US and Europe.

Sexual behavior and HIV among African adults

An early, influential study from Belgium and Rwanda reported scarcely believable rates of partner change among African men with AIDS or pre-AIDS. According to the study, the men had from 12 to 60 sexual partners per year, and 81 percent had visited sex workers at least once per month for the past two years.[31]

Other studies during 1984-88 found that such behavior was not characteristic of Africans with HIV infections. For example, a study in Kinshasa in 1987-88 found that 71 percent of 7,058 men working at a textile factory or bank and 99 percent of their 4,548 wives reported no non-marital partners in the past year. Only 2.3 percent of men reported more than five non-marital partners in the past year. Notably, men and women who reported no non-marital partners were found to have most of the HIV infections. Men who reported no non-marital partners had 143 (61 percent) of the 236 HIV infections in men, while men who reported more than five non-marital partners had only 13 (5.4 percent) of the infections in men. Women who reported no non-marital partners had 170 (97 percent) of the 175 HIV infections in women. Furthermore, more than 70 percent of HIV-positive wives had HIV-negative husbands. The study did not report the numbers of injections received by workers or wives, but noted that 'in Zaire patients who are ill always have high rates of receipt of injection with needles which may often have been re-used and not properly sterilized.'[32]

Another early study in Kigali, Rwanda, in 1988 found 25 women who were HIV-positive with HIV-negative husbands. Fifteen of these 25 women reported that their HIV-negative husband was their only lifetime sex partner.[33] The study team suggested that women had underreported their sexual activity.

Sex work and HIV

During 1984-88, some of the most influential research on risks for HIV infection in Africa was conducted through clinics treating sexually transmitted disease. During 1981-85, before anyone knew that AIDS was circulating in Kenya, researchers working through a special study clinic in Nairobi studied bacterial sexually transmitted disease among sex workers. Tests of stored blood from this study found 4 percent of sex workers to be HIV-positive in 1981, increasing precipitously to 82 percent in 1983, before falling back to 61 percent in 1985.[34] During this period, HIV prevalence in pregnant women attending antenatal clinics in Nairobi increased from 0 percent to 2 percent. Sex workers appeared to be leading Kenya's HIV epidemic.

Two subsequent studies that followed sex workers and male clients through Nairobi clinics that treated sexually transmitted disease observed high rates of HIV incidence.[35] During 1985-87, 67 percent of initially HIV-negative sex workers followed for an average of 18 months became HIV-positive. Similarly, 8 percent of male clients followed for an average of less than 4 months after seeking treatment for sexually transmitted disease became HIV-positive. Neither of these studies considered the possibility that blood tests and injections in study clinics transmitted HIV. Notably, sex workers who visited the study clinic more frequently, as well as sex workers who had genital ulcers (which were routinely treated with injections), were more likely to acquire HIV infections.

During the mid-1980s, Vachon,[36] Wyatt,[37] and others proposed that unsterile medical injections in Africa – especially injections to treat sexually transmitted disease – worked synergistically with sexual transmission to spread HIV infection among sex workers and clients. In 1985, Wycoff criticized one study that attributed high HIV prevalence among sex workers' clients to sexual transmission:[38]

> the reader is left to wonder if the risk factor for HTLV-III/LAV [HIV] spread in central Africa is prostitute exposures (e.g., heterosexual activity) or STD [sexually transmitted disease] clinic attendance (e.g., infected needles exposures). The implications of this uncertainty – economic, medical, and social – are very important to any evaluation of the AIDS epidemic in central Africa.

The hypothesis that clinics treating sexually transmitted disease infected sex workers and clients was not disproved – it was not even tested. At least part of the reason that studies failed to ask the right questions to trace HIV infections either to sex or to blood exposures was conflict of interest. Researchers working through clinics treating sexually transmitted disease could have been hurt by the finding that their clinics were spreading HIV. Nevertheless, clinic-based studies reporting high HIV prevalence and incidence among sex workers and clients were widely accepted to show a dominant role for heterosexual transmission in Africa's HIV epidemics.

Observed high rates of HIV prevalence among sex workers in Africa during 1984-88 contrasted sharply with findings from contemporaneous studies among sex workers in countries with concentrated epidemics. For example, in seven studies in Western Europe through 1987, less than 2 percent of a cumulative total of more than 2,700 sex workers were HIV-positive, and more than 60 percent of those who were HIV-positive were IDUs.[39] Few sex workers in Africa were IDUs, so that could not explain their high rates of HIV prevalence.

Early arguments that sex accounts for most HIV infections in Africa

In October 1985, WHO organized a workshop on AIDS in Central Africa, in Bangui, CAR. The memorandum from that workshop estimated that 80-90 percent of AIDS in African adults was from sexual transmission.[40] Through 1988, this position swept the field. It is useful to consider some of the assumptions, arguments, and evidence available through 1988 that supported this hypothesis.

During the 1980s, many AIDS experts supposed that differences between African vs. American and European AIDS epidemics could be explained by heterosexual behavior. For example, one 1987 analysis of Africa's AIDS epidemic generalized that 'most traditional African societies are promiscuous by Western standards. Promiscuity occurs both premaritally and postmaritally.'[41] Even if Africans were promiscuous relative to Americans or Europeans (which was soon disproved; see Chapter 7), and even if there were other factors that accelerated HIV transmission through heterosexual coitus in Africa, these differences would only support arguments that heterosexual coitus accounted for a higher proportion of HIV infections in Africa than in the US and Europe. However, that meant only an indeterminate percentage more than 3 percent – which was the proportion of cumulative AIDS cases among US adults attributed to heterosexual transmission through 1988. Such arguments did not support estimates that sex accounted for most infections in Africa.

Another common argument averred that the equal sex ratio among HIV-positive adults meant that most had contracted HIV through sex, but this was specious. Many diseases that infect men and women equally, such as colds and influenza, are not sexually transmitted.

In the 1980s – and onwards – the key argument supporting the hypothesis that sex accounted for most HIV infections in African adults had nothing to do with sex. Instead, the key argument was that blood exposures in health care did not account for many HIV infections, so that by elimination of other risks, infections in African adults must have come from heterosexual exposures. The next section considers evidence available through 1988 to assess the importance of HIV transmission through blood exposures.

Assessing generalized epidemics: Transmission through trace blood exposures

Exposures to HIV-contaminated equipment

Hundreds of studies during 1984-88 reported high HIV prevalence in patient populations in Africa and Haiti (Table 5.2). Whatever the reasons for these infections, they presented a threat to other patients when clinics reused instruments without sterilization.

During the 1980s, virtually everyone who was aware of healthcare practices in Africa reported that medical instruments were often reused without sterilization. For example, a 1987 study in Uganda observed that injections 'are often not given under aseptic conditions and themselves could theoretically be a vehicle of transmission.'[42] In Haiti, '...injections may be given by either medical personnel or piqurists (untrained injection doctors). Disposable needles and syringes are not readily available in Haiti, so needles and syringes may be reused without sterilization.'[43]

Moreover, studies during the 1980s showed that injections and other blood exposures were common.

HIV survival outside the body

In 1985, several French scientists who had helped to discover HIV reported its 'unusual stability' at room temperatures. For HIV kept in wet conditions, there was only a 'slight decrease' in its ability to grow in cell culture after seven days. Even when dried, some HIV remained infectious for seven days. The scientists advised that 'more safety precautions should be taken...in hospitals and by dentists...'[44]

Another study published in 1986 reported that some HIV (beginning with a concentrated solution with more HIV than would normally be found in blood) survived for more than 15 days in wet conditions and three or more days after drying.[45] In 1987, CDC reported results from its own studies showing that drying HIV for 'several hours' leaves 1 percent to 10 percent of HIV alive and infectious.[46]

Transmission risk through contaminated instruments

Studies during 1986-88 showed that almost everyone who received a transfusion of blood from an HIV-positive donor became infected.[47] However, this said little about the lower risk associated with exposures to very small amounts of blood, such as what might be found on medical instruments reused without sterilization.

To get some idea about the risk to pass HIV from patient to patient through contaminated instruments, people looked at IDUs who shared injection equipment. Studies through 1988 found high HIV prevalence among IDUs. But because IDUs get so many injections, this finding did not provide much information about the risk to transmit HIV through less frequent blood exposures during healthcare.

Another view of patients' risks to acquire HIV from contaminated instruments came from studies of healthcare workers after needlestick accidents. At least seven studies published in 1985-86 followed healthcare workers exposed to HIV through accidents, such as scratches or jabs with instruments that had just been used on HIV-infected patients. Combining information from these studies, only 3 (0.4 percent) of 818 workers developed HIV infections.[48] However, because most needlestick accidents are scratches that do not puncture the skin, this was not a reliable estimate of the risk to transmit HIV from one patient to others through injections and other skin-piercing procedures. Thus, other studies were required to measure the risks that people in Africa and in the Caribbean faced of acquiring HIV infection in healthcare settings, and to determine how much such risks contributed to HIV epidemics.

Early research linking HIV infections to health care in Africa

During 1984-88, the best research on blood exposures as risks for HIV infection in Africa came from Project SIDA (syndrome d'immuno deficience acquise), which was headquartered at Mama Yemo Hospital in Kinshasa. The governments of DRC, the US, and Belgium jointly sponsored Project SIDA. Researchers in Rwanda, Tanzania, Uganda, and other countries also asked about blood exposures as risks for HIV infection and reported useful information.

In 1985, Project SIDA tested inpatient and outpatient children aged 1-24 months and their mothers for HIV infection. Among 449 child-mother pairs, 44 children were HIV-positive. Surprisingly, 17 (39 percent) of the 44 HIV-positive children had mothers who were HIV-negative. Sixteen of the HIV-positive children with HIV-negative mothers were inpatients. These 16 children were an average of 11 months old and had received an average of 44 injections. Among children with HIV-negative mothers, 'medical injections seemed to be the most important risk factor for HIV seropositivity, followed by previous blood transfusions or hospital admission.' The study team noted, 'Injections are often administered in dispensaries which reuse needles and syringes yet may not adequately sterilize them.'[49]

In 1984-86, Lepage and colleagues conducted a similar study in Kigali, Rwanda, that produced similar results.[50] They tested the mothers of 76 children with AIDS aged 1-48 months. Eighteen (24 percent) of the mothers were HIV-negative. The 18 children with HIV-negative mothers had received an average of 23 injections, seven had been transfused, and eight had been previously hospitalized. Lepage and colleagues accepted that transfusions had infected some children, but did not want to accept that injections had done so as well. To see if there was some mistake, they retested 12 mothers who had previously tested HIV-negative. On this second test, three of 12 tested HIV-positive, leaving 15 (20 percent) of 76 HIV-positive children with HIV-negative mothers.

From this, the study team speculated that the HIV-negative test results for the other mothers may have been false-negatives as well. (Another possible – even likely – explanation for several mothers first testing negative and then positive is that they had contracted HIV infection from their children, possibly through breastfeeding, as later reported from Russia and Libya. See Chapter 9.) After raising doubts about evidence they did not like, Lepage and colleagues did not, either then or later, do the further research required to validate their doubts. The lack of resolution meant that Rwandan children were dying of unexplained AIDS, while medical researchers were satisfied to impugn evidence pointing to healthcare mistakes.

Thus, studies among children suggested that healthcare in Africa might be responsible for a lot of HIV infections among children. However, studies among children could not show how much HIV in adults was due to blood exposures. That could only be determined by studies among adults.

In mid-1984, Project SIDA tested 2,384 staff of Mama Yemo Hospital in Kinshasa.[51] One hundred and fifty-two (6.4 percent) were HIV-positive. Staff who reported injections in the past three years were 1.8 times more likely to be HIV-positive than those who reported no injections. During 1985-88, other studies in Rwanda, Tanzania, Uganda, and Zimbabwe asked about injections as risks for prevalent (existing) HIV infections in adults.[52] These studies found that adults who reported injections in recent years were 1.7 to 3.6 times more likely to be HIV-positive than those who reported no injections. Because most of the people in these studies reported injections, injections seemed to be linked to a lot of HIV infections.

However, the repeated finding that adults who had received injections in recent years were more likely to be HIV-positive did not necessarily show that injections transmitted HIV. Compared to people without HIV infections, people who were HIV-positive were more likely to be sick and therefore more likely to go for injections. This 'reverse causation' could explain some or all of the observed link between injections and prevalent HIV infection. Other study designs were needed to see how many HIV infections among adults were coming from injections and other invasive healthcare.

One way to minimize the problem of reverse causation is to find a group of HIV-negative people, and then follow and re-test them later to see who becomes HIV-positive, and ask everyone about risks. In 1986, Project SIDA re-tested 1,905 hospital employees who had been HIV-negative in 1984. In two years, 62 staff had acquired new HIV infections. Staff who reported one or more injections during those two years vs. staff who reported no injections were 1.53 times more likely to show up with an incident (new) infection.[53] However, the study team avoided the conclusion that injections were a risk for HIV infection. They reported that 6 of 62 people with incident infections had unspecified 'HIV-associated signs and symptoms' over the two years, and speculated that these six persons might have sought injections to treat HIV-related symptoms. After cutting these six persons out of the analysis, staff who reported injections were still 1.35 times more likely to show up with a new HIV infection. However, with the revised data, the observed greater risk to acquire HIV infection among those who reported injections was no longer 'significant.' To say the risk was no longer significant meant that the more frequent HIV infections among staff who reported injections may have been a statistical accident. In layman's terms, there was at least a 5 percent chance that injections did not infect any of the hospital staff.

Thus, during 1984-86, researchers had found HIV in children with HIV-negative mothers, and had followed HIV-negative adults to find that those who reported injections were more likely to acquire HIV infections. One interpretation of these findings is that injections and possibly other blood exposures caused a lot of HIV infection. Nevertheless, many researchers resisted this evidence with arguments that tests may have been bad, and that unwelcome findings may have been a statistical accident.

Considering the importance of the issue, and the suggestive evidence from these three early studies, one could have expected new studies of injections and other blood exposures as risks for incident HIV infection. These new studies could have been carefully designed to meet all doubts, so that health experts – and the public – would soon know if blood exposures during healthcare and cosmetic procedures were major contributors to Africa's HIV epidemics.

This did not happen. During 1985-88, only two other studies in Africa[54] and none in Haiti asked about injections as risks for incident HIV infections. The two studies (which have been mentioned earlier in this chapter) worked through clinics treating sexually transmitted disease in Nairobi, Kenya, to study HIV incidence in sex workers and clients. In these studies, the few sex workers and clients who reported injections or scarification outside the study clinics were not more likely to show up with new HIV infections. However, as already noted, neither study considered risks to transmit HIV through the much more common invasive procedures – injections and blood tests – in the study clinics. With their incomplete data, these two studies provide weak support for the position that blood exposures only rarely transmit HIV in Africa.

What about low HIV prevalence in children?

In the 1980s – and onwards – one of the most influential arguments that healthcare accounts for few HIV infections in Africa has been that low HIV prevalence in children (except young children with HIV-positive mothers) shows that injections seldom transmit HIV. Those who present this argument can cite many studies during 1984-88 (and later) that found few HIV infections in African children that could not be attributed to mother-to-child transmission. However, many other studies through 1988 (and later) have reported unexplained infections in children. For example, Rwanda's 1986 national survey found 4.2 percent of urban children aged 6-15 years to be HIV-positive.[55] And, as noted above, several hospital-based studies in 1984-86 found high percentages of HIV-positive children to have HIV-negative mothers.

Moreover, even in communities where children have few unexplained and possibly iatrogenic infections, this finding cannot be extrapolated to adults. Packard and Epstein have argued that the age-sex distribution of AIDS is not reliable evidence for sexual transmission:[56]

> ...if one looks at the age-sex distribution of tuberculosis [TB], one sees a similar pattern. Surely no one would argue that TB is a sexually transmitted disease....[I]t is generally noted that children in the age range from 4-14, for reasons which are not altogether clear, have a higher level of resistance to a number of diseases including TB. This period is often referred to as the 'golden years.' This phenomenon may in fact occur in AIDS.

Extending their argument, children vs. adults may be more able to resist HIV infection when exposed. Furthermore, children vs. adults may be treated in clinics where providers more often use sterile instruments, and where other patients are less often HIV-positive. Thus, low HIV prevalence in children does not show that adults are not contracting HIV during healthcare.

Assessing generalized epidemics: Transmission through blood transfusions

During 1984-88, at least 12 studies of risks for HIV infection in African adults and children (excluding studies among patients) asked about transfusions. Averaging results from these studies, transfusions appeared to have been responsible for about 5 percent of HIV infections.[57] In the late 1980s, AIDS experts generally accepted these results as an accurate measure of HIV infections from transfusions.

The contribution of transfusions to Africa's HIV epidemic was determined by the percentage of blood donors who were HIV-positive and the frequency of transfusions. In 1984-88, in the 12 African countries with the worst HIV epidemics and in Haiti, the median HIV prevalence among studies that tested blood donors for HIV ranged from a low of 3.0 percent in Zimbabwe to 18 percent in Rwanda and 20 percent from one study in Malawi (Table 5.2). Most African governments that answered a 1984 WHO questionnaire reported heavy reliance on paid and replacement donors.[58]

Some studies in Africa reported frequent transfusions, suggesting that doctors often transfused when other and safer treatments would suffice. For example, a 1984-85 study in Kinshasa found that 36 percent of inpatient children aged 2-14 years had been transfused (before their current hospitalization), and so had 14 percent of their healthy siblings.[59] People in sub-Saharan Africa (except South Africa) received an estimated 20 million transfusions in the 1980s[60] – equivalent to about 0.5 percent of the population receiving a transfusion each year. This shows a large increase from an estimated 12 million transfusions in the 1970s.

Risk for HIV among repeat blood donors

I have found no studies in Africa or Haiti during 1984-88 that asked about blood or plasma donation as a risk for HIV infection. However, reports from Spain[61] and Mexico in 1987-88 showed that donating plasma was a risk for HIV infection.

In 1986, shortly after the Mexican government ordered that all blood and plasma donations should be tested for HIV, tests found that 7 percent of paid donors were HIV-positive. Subsequently, tests of stored plasma from one private plasma-buying center identified 281 HIV-positive donors, including 62 repeat donors with new infections between June and October 1986.[62] Characteristically,[63]

> a paid donor would be a young man from a rural area who had migrated to one of the shanty towns that surround large cities...After hearing about the opportunity from a friend or family member, he would become a regular customer at one of the local blood banks or plasmapheresis centers, being paid to donate...as often as every 2 or 3 days. The more times he donated, the higher his risk became for becoming infected with HIV during the blood collection process.

After this study, Mexico banned blood sales from 1987. Subsequently, Mexico and the Panamerican Health Organization listed professional blood donors as a high-risk category for HIV infection in official statistics. WHO and African governments did not adopt this category.

AIDS control programs accept HIV transmission through healthcare in Africa

During the mid-1980s, many health experts in Europe and the US expected that healthcare practices in Africa would change to prevent HIV transmission to patients. For example, a *Lancet* editorial in 1987 identified 'the three main control activities' for HIV in Africa to be 'screening of donated blood, improvements in the use of sterile procedures by health workers, and health education designed to modify sexual behavior.' The editorial supposed that 'the first two measures are...at least in principle, moderately easy to achieve.'[64]

However, managers of the world's response to AIDS in Africa showed only a limited commitment to stop HIV transmission through healthcare. As already described, almost as soon as doctors in DRC and Rwanda started to test for HIV, they found HIV-positive children with HIV-negative mothers. Without investigations – asking where and when children had received care, and then testing others treated at the same facilities around the same time – it was not possible to determine the extent of the damage from infection control lapses, or to target interventions to the responsible facilities and procedures. There is no indication that international agencies or foreign health aid programs urged or offered to help with investigations. And there is no report that public health agencies in the affected countries investigated these or any other unexplained infections. Lack of investigations implicitly accepted continuing unknown numbers of nosocomial infections.

An important 1986 article on AIDS in Africa projected continuing unsafe practices: 'one cannot hope to prevent reuse of disposable injection equipment when many hospital budgets are insufficient for the purchase of antibiotics,' and 'one cannot expect public health officials to upgrade blood transfusion services to prevent HIV infection...'[65] The authors of that article include the heads of WHO's Global Programme on AIDS and later UNAIDS for most of the next 21 years. They expected – and subsequent HIV prevention programs accepted – that African clinics and hospitals would not reliably sterilize skin-piercing instruments, and would not test all transfused blood.

Initial but declining efforts to protect patients

The 1985 Bangui Workshop on AIDS in Central Africa discussed blood exposures as well as sex. The memorandum from the meeting noted, 'Epidemiological data show that non-sterile injections are responsible for a large proportion of AIDS cases in children,' and recommended, 'The public must be warned of the risk of AIDS transmission, especially through injections or scarifications carried out with equipment that is not disinfected and is re-used, both in modern medicine and in traditional medicine.'[66]

From 1986, WHO established the Global Programme on AIDS (initially named the Control Programme on AIDS). Along with an overwhelming emphasis on sexual behavior, early Global Programme documents discussed risks to transmit HIV in healthcare, and what to do about them. In 1986, the Global Programme's proposed outline for a national AIDS control program advised:[67]

> Prevention of [HIV] transmission through injections may require programmes to prevent reuse of single-use syringes/needles or methods to ensure reliable sterilization of reusable injection material. Programmes may also be directed towards sterilization of other instruments which pierce the skin or contact mucous membranes (e.g., scarifications, circumcision knives, ear-piercing).

In 1986, the Global Programme's proposed model budget for national AIDS prevention programs allocated 16 percent to a 'syringe/needle pilot project,' and 24 percent to test transfused blood for HIV. With this money, the Global Programme proposed that AIDS prevention programs provide sterilizers and self-destructing syringes, which could not be reused. Corresponding to this advice, Uganda in 1987 formulated a 5-year AIDS control plan, including, along with other components, infection control and blood safety. The program provided sterilizers, syringes, and needles for health centers and hospitals, and trained health staff in sterile techniques. [68]

The Global Programme's interest in infection control to protect patients was at its high point in 1986. After 1986, the Programme's documents show continuing awareness of widespread infection control lapses, but declining commitment to address them. For example, the Programme's 1988 guidelines for national AIDS programs urged governments to review infection control practices in formal and informal healthcare, but proposed no inputs or activities – aside from preparation of guidelines and professional training – to address infection control lapses.[69] Hence, for countries that recognized their epidemics early and asked for advice in 1986, the Global Programme urged them to allocate substantial efforts and resources to improve infection control. For countries that asked for advice after 1986, the Programme was much less intent on promoting infection control.

Limited commitment to blood safety (i.e., safe blood transfusions)

Through early 1986, only two African countries – South Africa and Zimbabwe – reported routine screening of donor blood for HIV.[70] Limited donor support for safe blood transfusions is illustrated by Project SIDA's activities in Kinshasa.

Project SIDA, headquartered at Mama Yemo Hospital, began using HIV tests in research in 1984. Not until two years later, in November 1986, did the project help the hospital to begin screening transfused blood for HIV. Even then, 'due to the lack of trained staff, ELISAs [testing] could be done only during the day.'[71] During the night, doctors continued to give emergency transfusions with untested fresh blood from someone who was available. This situation – testing during the day, but not at night – continued for 6 months. (Project SIDA took advantage of this situation to see what happened to people transfused with HIV-positive blood. By testing blood samples after blood had already been transfused, the Project identified 90 people who were HIV-negative when they entered the hospital, but who received HIV-positive blood. All or almost all patients – records were unreliable – given HIV-contaminated blood acquired HIV infections, and they were more likely to die over the following year than patients given HIV-negative blood.)

Like Project SIDA, WHO accepted transfusion of HIV-contaminated blood in Africa. In 1986, an expert committee organized by WHO recommended that countries should consider whether or not to test blood for HIV 'in the context of their overall health programmes and the availability of human and material resources.'[72] In 1987, the Programme Committee of WHO's Executive Board recommended transfusion of untested blood for an indefinite period:[73]

...in many developing countries...if one excluded all those who suffered from various tropical and parasitic diseases and hepatitis, as well as those who harboured HIV, the reservoir of potential safe donors would be substantially depleted. The cost of the necessary screening procedures to ensure the safety of the blood being donated was prohibitive...a pragmatic approach had to be followed in these countries to improve the situation progressively...

Initially, large budgets were required for new laboratories to test for HIV. In 1987, relatively low-cost rapid tests became available. From 1987, the Commission of European Communities (which later became the European Union) provided aid for blood safety in nine African countries.[74] Despite some improvements, progress was constrained by lack of money and commitment. In 1988, the Global Progamme on AIDS together with the League of Red Cross and Red Crescent Societies began the Global Blood Safety Initiative.[75] This initiative soon produced good plans to stop HIV transmission through blood transfusions, but these plans subsequently did not receive the support required to do so (Chapter 9).

Increasing but limited attention to protect healthcare workers

Whereas the Global Programme's attention to patients' risks fell over time, its attention to healthcare workers' risks increased. The Programme's first proposal for national AIDS control programs, prepared in 1986, does not mention healthcare workers' risks to acquire HIV from patients.[76] Two years later, the Global Programme's 1988 'Guidelines for nursing management of people infected with human immunodeficiency virus (HIV)' recommended infection control to protect both nurses and patients.[77] From 1987, the government of Uganda addressed healthcare-worker safety through short-term training and through the provision of gloves and other protective wear, 'especially for midwives and traditional birth attendants.' However, 'the gap between demand and supply remains wide...'[78] The situation for healthcare workers in Uganda was better than in most African countries.

Competing priorities to extend invasive healthcare

During the 1980s, WHO, UNICEF, and foreign donors were heavily committed to programs to extend immunizations for children and prenatal and delivery care for women. Such vertical programs (that focused on specific interventions) generated incentives to overlook systemic issues such as infection control. For managers and staff of vertical programs, concerns about infection control threatened their efforts to extend interventions as fast as possible at the lowest possible cost.

Among vertical programs, the Expanded Programme on Immunization (EPI) paid the most attention to infection control. As EPI's managers struggled to expand coverage in Africa, the surfacing of the AIDS epidemic forced them to reconsider injection practices. In 1986, an EPI policy document observed, 'Countries which for many years have tolerated the use of unsterile techniques for immunization and other injections are now faced with rising concerns about the risks which such practices entail.'[79]

The comment applies as well to EPI, WHO, and UNICEF managers. EPI decisions during 1985-88 provide a good example of the tension between vertical programs and infection control.

A 1985 meeting of WHO and UNICEF Regional Directors noted only 20 percent coverage of EPI immunizations in the Africa region, and asked for new initiatives to reach full coverage by 1990.[80] The report from the meeting did not mention HIV. Subsequently, WHO's Regional Committee for Africa declared 1986 to be African Immunization Year. During 1986, EPI delivered 62 million immunizations in Africa.[81]

A 1986 EPI report noted that 'the practice of multiple immunizations with a single needle and syringe (or with multiple needles and a single syringe) still occurs in immunization programmes,' and exhorted '*These practices must be stopped* [emphasis in original] and the "each child – one sterile syringe – one sterile needle" rule meticulously followed.'[82] However, another 1986 WHO and UNICEF document left a loophole for BCG immunization: 'The same syringe and needle are often used to administer BCG, but the only acceptable practice here is to flame the needle between injections.'[83]

Although EPI managers asked for safe injections, they did not insist. In 1987, a 'Joint WHO/UNICEF statement on immunization and

AIDS' envisioned a choice between unsafe injections for immunization and no immunizations: 'The potential for spread of HIV infection in childhood immunization sessions is low even where sterilization practices are below standard,' while 'Immunization programmes in developing countries are now preventing almost a million deaths a year...' Having posed this choice, without considering safe injections as a third option, WHO and UNICEF opted for unsafe immunizations: 'Halting immunization efforts because of the fear of AIDS would increase deaths among children, while doing little to stop HIV transmission.'[84]

Mann et al. in Kinshasa attributed many HIV infections in children to medical injections, but they pulled their punches when it came to immunizations. They argued from their data that 'childhood vaccination...was not associated with HIV seropositivity.'[85] This was a weak argument. Because only about 1 in 10 injections were immunizations, and because most children had received injections for immunization, it would have been difficult from their data to see a link between immunizations and HIV infection even if immunizations had infected several of the 44 HIV-positive children in their study. In 1988, Lepage and colleagues similarly asserted: 'The risk of HIV contamination [through immunization injections] is low if any, and should not compromise the immense benefit that wide-spread immunization campaigns have on children's health.'[86]

By October 1988, EPI had increased immunization coverage among African children to 56 percent for BCG, 40 percent for measles, and 38 percent for three doses of DPT (diphtheria, pertussis, tetanus), and 23 percent of pregnant women received two doses of tetanus vaccine.[87] On the other hand, limited commitment to safe injections brought limited results. In 1988, EPI's Global Advisory Group reported: 'The 1986 recommendation of a single sterile needle and syringe is now widely adopted as national EPI policy but is proving hard to realize in the field.'[88]

African public awareness and response to HIV risks in blood exposures

Some early AIDS prevention programs warned the African public about risks from unsafe injections. These warnings very likely had the biggest impact in countries with the worst epidemics, where people were aware of AIDS deaths. In Uganda, for example, many people kept syringes at home, which they brought to clinics when they wanted an injection. During the 1980s, Africans alert to risks no doubt found other ways to reduce their blood exposures during healthcare and cosmetic services. However, I have found little information about such practices at that time.

Despite some warnings, public health programs provided limited and often misleading information about risks. In at least one instance, too much public awareness of risks was considered a problem by public health managers. In 1988, public health mangers in Uganda linked a slowdown in the expansion of the EPI program to mothers' worries about the safety of reused glass syringes. Rather than responding positively to mothers' concerns by shifting to single-use equipment, public health managers reported that 'radio messages about AIDS in Uganda have been modified to ensure that parents are aware of the safety of immunizations.'[89] Ironically, other actions by EPI staff show they agreed with Ugandan mothers that injections with reused glass syringes were not safe. Already by 1987, EPI staff had initiated efforts to shift EPI injections to auto-destruct syringes that would break after one use (see Chapter 9).

1988 consensus on risks for HIV in generalized epidemics

From 1984, as soon as tests for HIV infection came available, researchers in Africa began to study the possibility that blood exposures in healthcare transmitted HIV. This was a far cry from what had happened after tests for hepatitis B infection were developed at the end of the 1960s – through 1988, no study had reported information on medical injections as risks for hepatitis B infection in African children.

Even so, research on risks for HIV infection did not resolve key questions. After several early studies published unwelcome results suggesting that injections accounted for a lot of HIV infections in African children and adults, there were no follow-up studies to confirm or refute these results. Instead, researchers avoided the issue. In 1988, leaders of the world's response to Africa's AIDS epidemic acknowledged that 'The role of certain practices in traditional and Western medicine, such as the reuse of needles, razor blades, or other instruments, in the spread of HIV infection has not been well documented...'[90]

In 1988, WHO asked a panel of experts to estimate the proportions of HIV infections in Africa and the Caribbean from all of the various routes of transmission. The panel estimated that heterosexual partners accounted for 80 percent of infections, mother-to-child transmission for 10.8 percent, blood transfusions for 6 percent, MSMs and IDUs for 1.6 percent, and medical injections and other blood exposures for 1.6 percent.[91] If these and other similar estimates had been recognized as hypotheses – which they were – they could have guided and stimulated research to prove or to disprove them. But this did not happen. Instead, the scientific community treated such estimates as established facts. For example, an editorial in the *Lancet* in 1988 misrepresented available evidence to claim that[92]

> ...epidemiological studies have shown that transfusion of HIV-infected blood or the use of unsterile needles or other skin-piercing instruments within the health system or as part of traditional healing (or other) practices can account for only a small proportion of HIV infections [in Africa].

From 1988, funders, journals, and colleagues accepted that researchers looking at risks for HIV infection in Africa did not have to ask about medical injections or other blood exposures in healthcare or cosmetic services. For example, a 1988 review of AIDS in sex workers did not mention risks of contracting HIV from unsterile medical instruments in Africa or elsewhere – but did note that sex workers who were IDUs in the US and Europe might contract HIV infections from needles and syringes reused to inject illegal drugs.[93]

From 1988, the consensus also released HIV prevention programs in countries with generalized epidemics from having to do anything about routine lapses in standard precautions in healthcare. As far as AIDS experts were concerned, it was none of their business.

---

[1] Chin J, Mann JM. 'The global patterns and prevalence of AIDS and HIV infection', *AIDS*, 1988, 2 (suppl 1): S247-52. p. S250.

[2] Sato PA, Chin J, Mann JM. 'Review of AIDS and HIV infection: Global epidemiology and statistics', *AIDS*, 1989, 3 (suppl 1): S301-7.

[3] CDC. *HIV/AIDS Surveillance Report: AIDS cases reported through December 1988.* Atlanta: CDC, 1989.

[4] Chin J, Mann JM. 'The global patterns'. p. S250.

[5] Sato PA et al. 'Review of AIDS and HIV infection'. p. S304; Chin J, Sato PA, Mann JM. 'Projections of HIV infections and AIDS cases to the year 2000', *Bull WHO*, 1990, 68: 1-11.

[6] World Bank. *African Development Indicators 1998/99*. Washington DC: World Bank, 1998.

[7] Table 5.1, WHO's estimates for HIV prevalence are from: Sato PA et al. 'Review of AIDS and HIV infection'.

[8] Table 5.1, reports from surveys, by country, are as follows: *Cote d'Ivoire* – Benoit SN, Gershy-Damet GM, Coulibaly A, et al. 'Seroprevalence of HIV infection in the general population of the Cote d'Ivoire, West Africa', *J Acquir Immune Defic Syndr*, 1990, 2: 1193-6; *Guinea-Bissau* – Piedade J, Venenno T, Prieto E, et al. 'Longstanding presence of HIV-2 infection in Guinea-Bissau (West Africa)', *Acta Trop*, 2000, 76: 119-24; *CAR and Congo* – Merlin M, Josse R, Trebucq A, et al. 'Surveillance epidemiologique du syndrome d'immunodepression acquise dans six etats d'Afrique Centrale', *Med Trop*, 1988, 48: 381-9; *Burundi* – Ministry of Health (Burundi). 'Surveillance Epidemiologique du VIH/SIDA/MST', unpublished document, Ministry of Health, 1992, reported in: US Census Bureau. *HIV/AIDS Surveillance Data Base, June 2003 release*. Washington, DC: US Census Bureau, 2003; *Rwanda*: Bizimungu C, Ntilivamunda A, Tahimana M, et al. 'Nationwide community-based serological survey of HIV-1 and other human retrovirus infections in a Central African country', *Lancet*, 1989, i: 941-3; *Uganda* – Kangeya-Kayondo JF, Amaana A, Naamara W. 'Anti-HIV seroprevalence in adult rural populations of Uganda and its implications for preventive strategies', 5th *Int Conf AIDS*, Montreal 4-6 June 1989, poster TAP 11 (the US Census Bureau's *HIV/AIDS Surveillance Data Base, June 2003 release*, reports data from this abstract that are not in the published abstract); Naamara W. 'Official Release of the National Serosurvey for Human Immunodeficiency Virus (HIV) in Uganda', unpublished letter to Minister of Health (Uganda), 1990, reported in: US Census Bureau. *HIV/AIDS Surveillance Data Base, June 2003 release*.

[9] Table 5.1, HIV prevalence in women attending urban antenatal clinics in Guinea-Bissau is from: US Census Bureau. *HIV/AIDS Surveillance Data Base, June 2003 release*. For other countries, see the Statistical Annex in this book for sources and for an explanation of the data in this column.

[10] Desmyter J, Goubau P, Chamaret S, et al. 'Anti-LAV/HTLV-III in Kinshasa mothers in 1970 and 1980 [abstract]', 2nd *Int Conf AIDS*, Paris 23-25 June 1986, abstract s17g.

[11] Nzilambi N, De Cock KM, Forthal DN, et al. 'The prevalence of infection with human immunodeficiency virus over a 10-year period in rural Zaire', *N Eng J Med*, 1988, 318: 276-9.

[12] Merlin M et al. 'Surveillance epidemiologique'.

[13] Musinguzi J. 'Women and AIDS: Are women at increased risk and what are the implications?' *East Afr Med J*, 1993, 70: 245-8; Mugerwa RD, Marum LH, Serwadda D. 'Human immunodeficiency virus and AIDS in Uganda', *East Afr Med J*, 1996, 73: 20-6.

[14] Berkley S, Naamara W, Okware S, et al. 'AIDS and HIV infection in Uganda – Are more women infected than men?', *AIDS*, 1990, 4: 1237-42.

[15] Killewo J, Nyamuryekunge K, Sandstrom A, et al. 'Prevalence of HIV-1 infection in the Kagera Region of Tanzania: A population-based study', *AIDS*, 1990; 4: 1081-5.

[16] US Census Bureau. *HIV/AIDS Surveillance Data Base, June 2003 release.*

[17] Sato PA et al. 'Review of AIDS and HIV infection'. p. S304.

[18] Simoes EAF, Babu PG, John TJ, et al. 'Evidence for HTLV-III infection in prostitutes in Tamil Nadu (India)', *Indian J Med Res*, 1987, 85: 335-8.

[19] Beyrer C. *War in the Blood: Sex, politics and AIDS in Southeast Asia.* London: Zed Books, 1998.

[20] Wright NH, Vanichseni S, Akarasewi P, et al. 'Was the 1988 HIV epidemic among Bangkok's injecting drug users a common source outbreak?', *AIDS*, 1994, 8: 529-32.

[21] Pape JW, Liautaud B, Thomas F, et al. 'The acquired immunodeficiency syndrome in Haiti', *Ann Intern Med*, 1985, 103: 674-8.

[22] N'Galy B, Ryder RW. 'Epidemiology of HIV infection in Africa', *J Acquir Immune Defic Syndr*, 1988, 1: 551-8.

[23] Van de Perre P, Clumeck N, Carael M, et al. 'Female prostitutes: A risk group for infection with human T-cell lymphotropic virus type III', *Lancet*, 1985, ii: 524-7.

[24] Mann JM, Francis H, Quinn TC, et al. 'HIV seroprevalence among hospital workers in Kinshasa, Zaire', *JAMA*, 1986, 256: 3099-102.

[25] Ryder RW, Ndilu M, Hassig SE, et al. 'Heterosexual transmission of HIV-1 among employees and their spouses at two large businesses in Zaire', *AIDS*, 1990, 4: 725-32.

[26] Melbye M, Njelesani EK, Bayley A, et al. 'Evidence for heterosexual transmission and clinical manifestations of human immunodeficiency virus infection and related conditions in Lusaka, Zambia', *Lancet*, 1986, ii: 1113-15.

[27] UNAIDS, WHO. *Cote d'Ivoire: Epidemiological Fact Sheets on HIV/AIDS and Sexually Transmitted Infections, 2000 update.* Geneva: WHO, 2000; similar UNAIDS' *Fact Sheets* for other countries, except that for Haiti the data are from the 2002 update.

[28] US Census Bureau. *HIV/AIDS Surveillance Data Base, June 2003 release.*

[29] CDC. 'Acquired immunodeficiency syndrome (AIDS) weekly surveillance report – United States, 31 December 1984'. Atlanta: CDC, 1984.

[30] Johnson AM, Laga M. 'Heterosexual transmission of HIV', *AIDS*, 1988, 2 (suppl 1): S49-56.

[31] Clumeck N, Carael M, Rouvroy D, et al. 'Heterosexual promiscuity among African patients with AIDS [letter]', *N Eng J Med*, 1985, 313: 182.

[32] Ryder RW et al. 'Heterosexual transmission of HIV-1'. p. 729.

[33] Allen S, Tice J, Van de Perre P, et al. 'Effect of serotesting with counselling on condom use and seroconversion among HIV discordant couples in Africa', *BMJ*, 1992, 304: 1605-9.

[34] Piot P, Plummer FA, Rey M-A, et al. 'Retrospective seroepidemiology of AIDS virus infection in Nairobi populations', *J Infect Dis*, 1987, 155: 1108-12.

[35] Plummer FA, Simonsen JN, Cameron DW, et al. 'Cofactors in male-female sexual transmission of human immunodeficiency virus type 1', *J Infect Dis*, 1991, 163: 233-9; Cameron DW, Simonsen JN, D'Costa LJ, et al. 'Female to male transmission of human immunodeficiency virus type 1: Risk factors for seroconversion in men', *Lancet*, 1989; ii: 403-7.

[36] Vachon F, Coulaud JP, Katlama C. 'Epidemiologie actuelle du syndrome d'immunodeficit acquis en dehors des groupes a risque', *Presse Med*, 1985, 14: 1949-50.

[37] Wyatt HV. 'Injections and AIDS', *Trop Doctor*, 1986, 16: 97-8.

[38] Wykoff RF. 'Female-to-male transmission of AIDS agent [letter]', *Lancet*, 1985; ii: 1017-18.

[39] Cohen JB, Wofsy C, Gill P, et al. 'Antibody to human immunodeficiency virus in female prostitutes', *MMWR*, 1987, 36: 157-61.

[40] WHO. 'Workshop on AIDS in Central Africa, Bangui, Central African Republic, 22-25 October 1985.' Geneva: WHO, 1986. Doc. no. WHO.CDS.AIDS/85.1.

[41] Hrdy DB. 'Cultural practices contributing to the transmission of human immunodeficiency virus in Africa', *Rev Infect Dis*, 1987, 9: 1109-19. p. 1112.

[42] Konde-Lule JK, Berkley SF, Downing R. 'Knowledge, attitudes and practices concerning AIDS in Ugandans', *AIDS*, 1989, 3: 513-18. p. 517.

[43] Pape JW, Liautaud B, Thomas F, et al. 'The acquired immunodeficiency syndrome in Haiti', *Ann Intern Med*, 1985, 103: 674-8. p. 677.

[44] Barre-Sinoussi F, Nugeyre MT, Chermann JC. 'Resistance of AIDS virus at room temperature [letter]', *Lancet*, 1985; ii: 721-2.

[45] Resnick L, Veren K, Salahuddin Z, et al. 'Stability and inactivation of HTLV-III/LAV under clinical and laboratory conditions', *JAMA*, 1986, 255: 1887-91.

[46] CDC. 'Recommendations for prevention of HIV transmission in health-care settings', *MMWR*, 1987, 36 (suppl 2S): 3S-18S.

[47] Berglund O, Beckman S, Grillner L, et al. 'HIV transmission by blood transfusion in Stockholm 1979-85: nearly uniform transmission from infected donors', *AIDS*, 1988, 2: 51-4; Colebunders R, Ryder R, Francis H, et al. 'Seroconversion rate, mortality, and clinical manifestations associated with the receipt of a human immunodeficiency virus-infected blood transfusion in Kinshasa, Zaire', *J Infect Dis*, 1991, 164: 450-6.

[48] Wormser GP, Joline C, Sivak SL, et al. 'Human immunodeficiency virus infections: considerations for health care workers', *Bull New York Acad Med*, 1988, 64: 203-15.

[49] Mann JM, Francis H, Davachi F, et al. 'Risk factors for human immunodeficiency virus seropositivity among children 1-24 months old in Kinshasa, Zaire', *Lancet*, 1986, ii: 654-7. p. 656.

[50] Lepage P, Van de Perre P, Carael M, et al. 'Are medical injections a risk factor for HIV in children?', *Lancet*, 1986, ii: 1103-4; Lepage P, Van de Perre P. 'Nosocomial transmission of HIV in Africa: What tribute is paid to contaminated blood transfusions and medical injections?', *Infect Control Hosp Epidemiol*, 1988, 9: 200-3.

[51] Mann JM et al. 'HIV seroprevalence among hospital workers'.

[52] Van de Perre P, Carael M, Nzaramba D, et al. 'Risk factors for HIV seropositivity in selected urban-based Rwandese adults', *AIDS*, 1987, 1: 207-11; Killewo J et al. 'Prevalence of HIV-1 infection in the Kagera Region of Tanzania'; Konde-Lule JK et al. 'Knowledge, attitudes and practices'; Bassett MT, Latif AS, Katzenstein DA, et al. 'Sexual behavior and risk factors for HIV infections in a group of male factory workers who donated blood in Harare, Zimbabwe', *J Acquir Immune Defic Syndr*, 1992, 5: 556-9.

[53] N'Galy B, Ryder RW, Bila K, et al. 'Human immunodeficiency virus infection among employees in an African hospital', *N Eng J Med*, 1988, 319: 1123-7.

[54] Plummer FA et al. 'Cofactors in male-female sexual transmission'; Cameron DW et al. 'Female to male transmission', *Lancet*, 1989, ii: 403-7.

[55] Bizimungu C et al. 'Nationwide community-based serological survey'.

[56] Packard RM, Epstein P. 'Epidemiologists, social scientists, and the structure of medical research on AIDS in Africa', *Soc Sci Med*, 1991, 33: 771-83. p. 780.

[57] Gisselquist D, Potterat JJ, Brody S, et al. 'Let it be sexual: How health care transmission of AIDS in Africa was ignored', *Int J STD AIDS*, 2003, 14: 148-61.

[58] WHO. 'Blood and Blood Products: Report by the Director-General, 14 January 1987.' Geneva: WHO, 1987. Doc. no. EB79/7, Add. 1.

[59] Mann JM, Francis H, Davachi F, et al. 'Human immunodeficiency virus seroprevalence in pediatric patients 2 to 14 years of age at Mama Yemo Hospital, Kinshasa, Zaire', *Pediatrics*, 1986, 78: 673-7.

[60] Schneider WH, Drucker E. 'Blood transfusions in the early years of AIDS in sub-Saharan Africa', *Am J Pub Health*, 2006, 96: 984-94.

[61] Navarro V, Roig P, Nieto A, et al. 'A small outbreak of HIV infection among commercial plasma donors [letter]', *Lancet*, 1988, ii: 42.

[62] Avila C, Stetler HC, Sepulveda J, et al. 'The epidemiology of HIV transmission among paid plasma donors, Mexico City, Mexico', *AIDS*, 1989, 3: 631-3.

[63] del Rio C, Sepulveda J. 'AIDS in Mexico: Lessons learned and implications for developing countries', *AIDS*, 2002, 16: 1445-57. pp. 1446-7.

[64] 'AIDS in Africa', *Lancet*, 1987, ii: 192-4. p. 193.

[65] Quinn TC, Mann JM, Curran JW, Piot P. 'AIDS in Africa: An epidemiologic paradigm', *Science*, 1986, 234: 955-63. p. 962.

[66] WHO. 'Workshop on AIDS in Central Africa, Bangui, Central African Republic, 22-25 October 1985.' Geneva: WHO, 1986. Doc. no. WHO.CDS.AIDS/85.1. pp. 11, 12.

[67] WHO. 'Global WHO Strategy for the Prevention and Control of Acquired Immunodeficiency Syndrome: Projected Needs for 1986-1987.' Geneva: WHO, 1986. Doc. no. AIDS/CPA86.2. pp. 22, 27.

[68] Okware SI. 'Towards a national AIDS-control programme in Uganda', *West J Med*, 1987, 147: 726-9.

[69] WHO. 'Guidelines for the development of a national AIDS prevention and control program', WHO AIDS series 1. Geneva: WHO, 1988. Available at: http://whqlibdoc.who.int/aids/WHO_AIDS_1.pdf (accessed 4 September 2007).

[70] WHO. 'Blood and Blood Products'.

[71] Colebunders R et al. 'Seroconversion rate, mortality, and clinical manifestations'. p. 450.

[72] 'Acquired Immune Deficiency Syndrome (AIDS): WHO meeting and consultation on the safety of blood products', in: Petricciani JC, Gust ID, Hoppe PA, et al. (eds), *The Safety of Blood and Blood Products*. Geneva: WHO, 1987. pp. 355-359. The quote is from page 356.

[73] WHO. 'Blood and Blood Products: Report by the Programme Committee of the Executive Board.' Geneva: WHO, 1987. Doc. no. EB79/7. pp. 4-5.

[74] Fleming AF. 'HIV and blood transfusion in sub-Saharan Africa', *Transfu Sci*, 1997, 18: 167-79.

[75] WHO. 'Report of the Global Blood Safety Initiative Meeting, Geneva, 16-17 May 1988.' Geneva: WHO, 1988. Doc. no. WHO/GPA/DIR/88.9.

[76] WHO. 'Global WHO Strategy'.

[77] WHO. 'Guidelines for nursing management of people infected with human immunodeficiency virus (HIV)', WHO AIDS series 3. Geneva: WHO, 1988. Available at: http://whqlibdoc.who.int/aids/WHO_AIDS_3.pdf (accessed 4 September 2007).

[78] Okware SI. 'Towards a national AIDS-control programme in Uganda'. p. 729.

[79] WHO. 'Immunization Policy.' Doc. no. WHO/EPI/GEN/86/7 Rev 1. Geneva: WHO, 1986. p. 8.

[80] WHO. 'Final Report, WHO/UNICEF Regional Directors' Consultation, Brazzaville 3-4 September 1985.' Geneva: WHO, 1985. Doc. no. AFR/EXM/10.

[81] WHO. 'Report of the Expanded Programme on Immunization, Global Advisory Group meeting, Washington DC, 9-13 November 1987.' Geneva: WHO, 1988. Doc. no. WHO/EPI.GEN/88.1.

[82] LaForce FM. 'Immunization of children infected with human immunodeficiency virus', Geneva: WHO, 1986. Doc. no. WHO/EPI/GEN/86/6 Rev. 1. p. 4.

[83] WHO. 'Selection of Injection Equipment for the Expanded Programme on Immunization', EPI Technical Series. Geneva: WHO, 1986. Doc. no. WHO/UNICEF/EPI.TS/86.2. p. 4.

[84] 'Expanded Programme on Immunization: Joint WHO/UNICEF statement on HIV and immunization', *Wkly Epidemiol Rec*, 1987, 62: 53-4. p. 53.

[85] Mann JM et al. 'Risk factors for human immunodeficiency virus seropositivity'. p. 656.

[86] Lepage P, Van de Perre P. 'Nosocomial transmission of HIV in Africa'. p. 203.

[87] WHO. 'Report of the Expanded Programme on Immunization Global Advisory Group Meeting, Abidjan, Cote d'Ivoire, 17-21 October 1988', Geneva: WHO, 1989. Doc. no. WHO/EPI/GEN/89.1.

[88] Ibid. p. 71.

[89] Berkley S, Weeks M, Barenzi J. 'Immunization and fear of AIDS [letter]', *Lancet*, 1990, i: 47-48.

[90] Piot P, Plummer FA, Mhalu FS, et al. 'AIDS: An international perspective', *Science*, 1988, 239: 573-9. p. 578.

[91] Chin J et al. 'Projections of HIV infections and AIDS cases'.

[92] 'AIDS in sub-Saharan Africa', *Lancet*, 1988, i: 1260-1. p. 1260.

[93] Day S. 'Prostitute women and AIDS: Anthropology', *AIDS*, 1988, 2: 421-8.

Chapter 6

THINGS GO BADLY WRONG, 1989-2007

By 1988, the world's public health experts had studied HIV and had settled on strategies to stop it. Knowledge of HIV led to dramatic slowing of epidemic expansion in some countries, but not in others. From 1989, new generalized epidemics emerged in Africa and Asia. New epidemics in relatively wealthy African countries became much worse than anything that had developed in the fifty or so years to 1981, when no one knew anything about AIDS or HIV.

Table 6.1: World overview of HIV epidemic expansion, 1988-2007

Epidemic type, region, country	HIV infections (1,000s)	
	1988[1]	2007[2]
Concentrated epidemics, of which:	2,500	6,700
North and South America	*2,000*	*2,800*
Western Europe	*500*	*760*
Eastern Europe and Central Asia	*†*	*1,600*
East Asia, Southeast Asia, South Asia, and Oceania	*†*	*1,400*
Middle East and North Africa	*†*	*100*
Generalized epidemics, of which:	2,500	25,000
Sub-Saharan Africa	*2,500*	*21,000*
Caribbean region (Haiti, 9 other small countries)	***	*300*
Asia and Oceania (Cambodia, India, Myanmar, Papua New Guinea, Thailand)	*†*	*3,500*
Total	5,100	32,000

* Included in the estimate for Africa.
† In 1988, WHO estimated 100,000 HIV infections in Asia, Central and Eastern Europe, the Middle East, and North Africa.
Sources: See references by column.

Concentrated epidemics

As of 1988, WHO estimated *circa* 2.5 million HIV infections in Pattern 1 epidemics in the Americas, Western Europe, Australia, and New Zealand, which was about half of all HIV infections in the world (Table 6.1). During 1989-2007, most new epidemics outside Africa developed as concentrated epidemics. In 2007, countries with concentrated epidemics accounted for an estimated 6.7 million infections – about one-fifth of HIV infections in the world. Estimated adult HIV prevalence varied across countries from near 0.01 percent (1 in 10,000), as in Bangladesh and Bulgaria, to 1.1-1.4 percent in Estonia, Moldova, Russia, and Ukraine (these estimates exceeding 1 percent may be too high).

Stabilizing old concentrated epidemics

Beginning from the early 1980s, most of the MSMs and IDUs who were infected or at risk in old concentrated epidemics progressively changed their behavior. By the early 1990s, an average HIV-positive person infected less than one other person in their life. Deaths matched or exceeded new infections. Most of the modest expansion in old concentrated epidemics during 1989-2007 occurred in South America.

During the 1980s, some AIDS experts hypothesized that concentrated epidemics in the US and Europe would progress naturally to generalized epidemics, as in Africa. This has not happened. In the US, Western Europe, Canada, and Australia, MSMs and IDUs accounted for 75-88 percent of cumulative adult and adolescent AIDS cases through mid- to end-2005, and the proportion attributed to heterosexual risk ranged from 7 percent to 16 percent (excluding persons born in countries with generalized epidemics).[3]

Although many HIV-positive bisexuals and IDUs have been heterosexually active, only a minority has infected heterosexual partners through sex, and subsequent heterosexual spread from these partners to others has been limited. Studies estimate that heterosexual transmission has been too slow to sustain HIV epidemics in the US[4] and Norway.[5] Although HIV 'leaks' into the general population, people who are neither IDUs nor MSMs on average die before passing HIV to anyone else.

IDUs drive new concentrated epidemics

While MSMs dominate most of the old concentrated epidemics, IDUs drive the new ones. The five largest new epidemics emerged in Russia (940,000 infections estimated in 2005), China (650,000 infections), Ukraine (410,000 infections), Vietnam (260,000 infections), and Indonesia (170,000 infections).[6]

HIV circulated among MSMs in Russia in the 1980s, but infections were rare. Through 1995, only 1,062 HIV infections had been detected, and only 7 were in IDUs.[7] From 1996, HIV infection took off among IDUs, and so did Russia's epidemic. For Russia and for all Eastern Europe through 2005, IDUs accounted for more than 80 percent of cumulative reported infections with information on risk.[8]

The first AIDS case in China was reported in 1985 from Yunnan Province near Myanmar. IDUs spread HIV throughout China, reaching all of China's 31 provinces by 1998. A 2002 assessment of China's HIV epidemic attributed 60-70 percent of infections to IDUs.[9] As of 2005, the Chinese government estimated that 650,000 people (less than 0.1 percent of adults) were living with HIV. At the same time, the government attributed 44 percent of infections to IDUs, 7 percent to MSMs, and 11 percent to blood or plasma donors and transfusions recipients.[10]

Vietnam's HIV epidemic similarly began in the 1980s. Through 1999, IDUs accounted for 88 percent of identified infections.[11] Indonesia's epidemic took off among IDUs in the late 1990s. During 1997-2001, HIV prevalence among IDUs in a rehabilitation center in Jakarta, the capital, increased from 0 percent to 48 percent.[12]

Are there other kinds of concentrated HIV epidemics?

Currently, UNAIDS and WHO classify HIV epidemics into three categories: generalized epidemics, in which HIV prevalence exceeds 1 percent in the general population; concentrated epidemics, in which prevalence exceeds 5 percent in at least one group, but is less than 1 percent in the general population; and low-level epidemics, in which HIV prevalence does not exceed 5 percent in any group.[13]

These categories extend the concept of a concentrated epidemic beyond MSMs and IDUs to include epidemics in which HIV infections concentrate in groups that are heterosexually promiscuous – especially women in sex work and clients. This poses an empirical question: does a small group of heterosexually promiscuous men and women account for most HIV infections in any country? This chapter and Chapter 7 present relevant evidence.

Futhermore, these categories obscure an important distinction. In the 1980s WHO recognized different sex ratios among those with HIV infections in Pattern 1 vs. Pattern 2 epidemics. Pattern 1 epidemics infected mostly men, while Pattern 2 epidemics afflicted women as often or more often than men. This distinction based on the sexual distribution of infections is lost if the category of concentrated epidemics is extended to include epidemics with high HIV prevalence in sex workers. If one is trying to understand differences among HIV epidemics, it is arguably important to use categories which preserve attention to vastly different sex ratios among HIV-positive people.

Thus, in this book, 'concentrated epidemics' refers to those in which infections concentrate in MSMs and/or IDUs, while 'generalized epidemics' refers to those in which HIV prevalence in women is greater than or comparable to prevalence in men. With these definitions, low-level epidemics may be low-level concentrated or generalized epidemics, depending on the proportion of infections in MSMs and IDUs and on the sex ratio among those who are infected. With these terms, there may also be mixed epidemics, where MSMs and IDUs account for a large minority of infections, but HIV also infects many non-IDU women.

Generalized epidemics in Africa

Whereas awareness of HIV led to limited growth of concentrated epidemics after 1988, awareness had less impact on generalized epidemics. During 1988-2007, the total number of HIV infections in generalized epidemics increased by an estimated 23 million – from 2.5 million to 25 million. Most of this increase occurred in Africa (Table 6.1 and Statistical Annex).

One of the difficulties in tracking generalized HIV epidemics over the years has been that official estimates of HIV prevalence have often been far off the mark. Consider Ethiopia. In 1994, WHO estimated that 2.5 percent of Ethiopian adults were HIV-positive. By 2000, UNAIDS reported that HIV prevalence had increased to 10.6 percent. In 2005, the Ethiopian government conducted a national survey – and found that only 1.6 percent of adults were infected![14]

During 2001-07, more than thirty governments of countries with generalized epidemics implemented national surveys of HIV infection. In these countries, estimates of HIV prevalence are on solid ground. As of early 2007, only a few countries with generalized epidemics and without surveys – especially Nigeria and Mozambique – have sufficient estimated infections that future surveys could have more than a small impact on regional and world estimates of HIV infections.

Through 2007, Africa's HIV epidemics took several paths. Many of the countries with the worst epidemics in 1988 showed little or no epidemic expansion, while terrible new epidemics emerged in Southern Africa. Outside of Southern Africa, the most serious new epidemics developed in three relatively wealthy countries in East and Central Africa (Kenya, Cameroon, and Gabon). At the same time, many African countries, including countries at war, continued to have only low-level generalized epidemics. The following subsections describe these different paths.

What happened to Africa's worst epidemics from 1988?

In 1988, WHO had identified 12 countries in Africa with at least 0.5 percent of the population infected (children and adults). Three of these 12 countries – Malawi, Zambia, and Zimbabwe – are in Southern Africa. Epidemics in these three countries developed into some of the worst in the world (see next subsection). In the remaining nine countries in Central Africa (CAR, Congo, and DRC), West Africa (Cote d'Ivoire and Guinea-Bissau), and East Africa (Burundi, Rwanda, Tanzania, and Uganda), HIV epidemics expanded more slowly or not at all during 1989-2007.

In 1988, these nine countries probably had roughly two-thirds of WHO's estimated 2.5 million infections in Africa. Through 2005, the estimated number of infections in these nine countries together increased, by a factor of about three, to 4.5 million. The figure for 2005 is close to accurate – it is based on national surveys in six of the nine countries with more than three-fourths of estimated infections. In 2006, the total population in these nine countries was 160 million, and the weighted average adult HIV prevalence was 5 percent.

Some countries did better than others. Results from Cote d'Ivoire's 1989 and 2005 national surveys showed adult HIV prevalence falling from 6 percent to 4.7 percent over 16 years. Even if errors in the 1989 survey (such as false positive tests) had inflated estimated prevalence, Cote d'Ivoire's epidemic likely grew little if at all after 1989. Similarly, national surveys in Rwanda in 1986 and 2005 found, respectively, 2.7 percent and 3.0 percent adult HIV prevalence, showing little epidemic expansion over 19 years. Burundi's national survey in 2002 reported 3.6

percent of adults to be HIV-positive, so that HIV prevalence may have doubled from roughly 2 percent in a 1989 survey. Although no national survey has been accomplished in DRC, sentinel surveys among women in urban antenatal clinics suggest stable or falling HIV prevalence from the late 1980s (see also the subsection on African wars, below).

More than half the estimated HIV infections in these nine countries are found in Tanzania and Uganda, with 1.4 million and 1 million infections, respectively, in 2005. In Tanzania, HIV prevalence fell from the late 1980s in heavily infected regions west of Lake Victoria. Surveys in Bukoba town, for example, found 24 percent of adults to be HIV-positive in 1987, but only 13 percent in 1996.[15] However, these reductions were offset by gains elsewhere, so that Tanzania's HIV prevalence increased from 1988 to 2007. Tanzania's first national survey in 2003 found 7.0 percent adult HIV prevalence, which is one of the highest rates outside Southern Africa.

In Uganda, several estimates based on the 1987-88 national survey suggest adult HIV prevalence of 7-10 percent, which may have been misleadingly high (see Chapter 5). Uganda's second and more complete national survey in 2004-05 reported 6.3 percent HIV prevalence in adults aged 15-59 years. For some years around 1990, Uganda probably had the highest HIV prevalence in Africa – but how high? In any case, Uganda's HIV prevalence in 2004-05 is one of the highest outside Southern Africa.

From the mid-1990s, many AIDS experts have presented Uganda as the country with the best success against HIV in Africa. For example, an article in *Science* in 2004 declared, 'Uganda has shown a 70 percent decline in HIV prevalence since the early 1990s...'[16] This and similar claims of success are based largely on data from selected urban antenatal clinics, where HIV prevalence often topped 20 percent during 1987-1996.[17] However, HIV prevalence in these clinics was not only far greater than in Uganda's rural population, but falling prevalence in these clinics also did not reflect what was happening in rural areas. For example, in 15 villages in rural Masaka west of Lake Victoria, adult HIV prevalence fell only modestly during 1989-99 from 7.8 percent to 6.4 percent.[18]

AIDS experts argue about whether Uganda's success was due to more condom use or to fewer sexual partners. These arguments ignore possible reductions in non-sexual transmission. From 1987 the government promoted infection control for AIDS prevention, and public awareness of risks with blood exposures energized public demands for safe injections. In any case, the presentation of Uganda as the county with the best success against AIDS in Africa overlooks other African countries with lower and/or falling HIV prevalence, such as Cote d'Ivoire, DRC, and Rwanda. As Tim Allen documents in a 2006 review, 'Interpretations of HIV/AIDS in Uganda have taken on lives of their own, in which evidence of all kinds plays a secondary role.'[19]

Across all nine countries in Central, East, and West Africa with the worst epidemics in 1988, HIV prevalence in the early 2000s was, of course, higher in women than in men. It was also much higher in urban than in rural populations. In the four countries for which we have data, HIV prevalence in women increased with wealth, and (less consistently) with education (Table 6.2). Rich, educated, urban women were several times more likely to be HIV-positive than poor, illiterate, rural men.

Table 6.2: Recent distribution of HIV infections in African countries* with the worst epidemics in 1988

Country, year of survey	HIV prevalence (%) in adults		HIV prevalence (%) in women by education			HIV prevalence (%) in women by wealth quintiles				
	Urban	Rural	None	Prim-ary	Secondary or higher	Low-est	2nd	3rd	4th	High-est
Cote d'Ivoire, 2005										
Women	7.4	5.5	5.2	8.2	7.0	3.6	3.8	6.5	8.0	8.8
Men	3.2	2.5								
Rwanda, 2005										
Women	8.6	2.6	3.3	2.8	6.4	2.6	2.2	3.6	3.4	6.5
Men	5.8	1.6								
Tanzania, 2003										
Women	12.0	5.8	5.8	8.1	9.3	2.8	4.6	6.8	10.9	11.4
Men	9.6	4.8								
Uganda, 2004-05										
Women	12.8	6.5	5.8	8.1	7.6	4.8	6.6	6.7	7.0	11.0
Men	6.7	4.7								

*All countries for which survey data are available.
Sources: See the Statistical Annex.

The world's worst epidemics in Southern Africa

Most of the countries in Southern Africa are wealthy by African standards. In the 1990s, per capita incomes in South Africa and Botswana were 10 times the average for the rest of sub-Saharan Africa.

Per capita incomes in Lesotho, Namibia, Swaziland, and Zimbabwe were several times averages for the rest of sub-Saharan Africa (excluding South Africa).[20]

In 1988, WHO estimated that more than 1 percent of the population (2 percent of adults) was HIV-positive in Malawi and Zambia, and more than 0.5 percent was HIV-positive in Zimbabwe. In Southern Africa, Mozambique is the only other county with evidence for substantial numbers of HIV infections through 1988. Surveys among adults in 10 cities in Mozambique in 1987 reported several percent HIV prevalence,[21] but most people lived in rural areas with lower prevalence.

The 50 South Africans recognized with AIDS through March 1987 were all white men with risks found in concentrated epidemics.[22] In 1988, HIV was just beginning to spread among South Africa's majority black population. In Natal Province of South Africa, HIV prevalence among black blood donors passed 0.1 percent in late 1988 and 0.2 percent in early 1989.[23] In Lesotho, none of more than 5,000 blood donors was HIV-positive in 1988.[24]

Figure 6.1: HIV prevalence in pregnant women* attending urban antenatal clinics, for nine countries in Southern Africa, 1985-2005

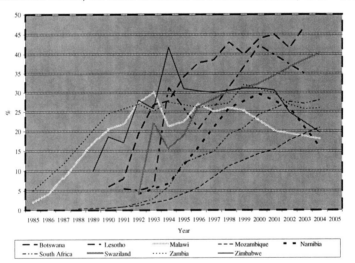

* Median HIV prevalence among selected (sentinel) urban antenatal clinics.
Source: WHO's epidemiological Fact Sheets on HIV/AIDS and sexually transmitted infections for various countries and years (see the Statistical Annex).

Throughout Southern Africa, HIV prevalence in pregnant women attending urban antenatal clinics soared in the early 1990s (Figure 6.1). High prevalence in Mozambique began after the civil war ended in 1992. Madagascar was the only exception. For reasons that are not well understood, Madagascar has sustained one of the lowest rates of adult HIV prevalence among African countries – estimated at 0.2 percent in 2005.

From 1988 to 2005, the number of HIV infections in nine countries in Southern Africa – Botswana, Lesotho, Malawi, Mozambique, Namibia, South Africa, Swaziland, Zambia, and Zimbabwe – increased from possibly around 300,000 to 10 million. Estimates for 2005 are based on recent national surveys in seven of the nine countries. As of 2005, these nine countries, with a seventh of Africa's population, accounted for almost half of Africa's HIV infections, and their weighted average adult HIV prevalence was 16 percent.

The explosion of the region's HIV epidemic occurred in the face of well-funded public health programs. By the early 1980s, the government of Botswana, with its own money from diamonds and with donor support, had constructed a public health post or clinic within 15 kilometers of more than 90 percent of the population, and provided mobile services to reach the rest.[25] In the 1990s, the South African government expanded public health services to the black majority. During 1990-95, public expenditures on health in the nine countries in Southern Africa with the emerging worst AIDS epidemics ranged from 1.9 percent to 4.6 percent (with a median of 3.0 percent) of gross domestic product, compared to an average of less than 1.3 percent for the rest of Africa.[26]

During the 1990s, countries in the region implemented HIV prevention programs guided by international advice. In 2001, the Harvard AIDS Institute honored Botswana's President Festus Mogae with its Leadership Award. Harvard's publicity surrounding the event lauded Botswana's response to the epidemic.[27] In 2003, an international team judged that Swaziland's response to the AIDS epidemic 'has been in accordance with international norms, and indeed in many places has gone beyond them…Swaziland was one of the earliest countries to make mention of HIV in its national development plans…'[28]

From the late 1990s, critics have attacked the South African government for opposing the use of antiretroviral drugs to reduce mother-to-child HIV transmission, and later to treat people with AIDS. Thabo Mbeki, the president of South Africa from 1999, has been criticized for his dialogue with denialists, who say HIV does not cause AIDS. These controversies focus on treatment, and began after HIV had already overrun the country. During the 1990s,[29] and continuing, programs to prevent HIV infections among adults followed international advice, promoting sexual behavior change, condoms, and treatment of sexually transmitted disease.

Even within relatively wealthy countries in Southern Africa, women's HIV prevalence often increased with wealth (but generally did not increase with education). As in most countries in Africa, women were more heavily infected than men. However, in some countries, there was little difference between urban and rural adults (Table 6.3).

Table 6.3: Distribution of HIV infections in Southern African countries* with the worst current epidemics

Country, year of survey	HIV prevalence (%) in adults		HIV prevalence (%) in women by education			HIV prevalence (%) in women by wealth quintiles				
	Urban	Rural	None	Prim-ary	Secondary or higher	Low-est	2nd	3rd	4th	High-est
Lesotho, 2004										
Women	33.0	24.3	30.4	26.5	26.0	19.6	27.9	25.5	27.3	28.9
Men	22.0	18.6								
Malawi, 2004										
Women	18.0	12.5	13.6	12.8	15.1	10.9	10.3	12.7	14.6	18.0
Men	16.3	8.8								
Zambia, 2001-02										
Women	26.3	12.4								
Men	19.2	8.9								
Zimbabwe, 2005-06										
Women	21.6	20.8	20.0	22.4	20.4	17.7	21.1	22.7	26.8	17.1
Men	15.7	13.8								

* All countries for which survey data are available.
Sources: See the Statistical Annex.

Other Africa countries with severe epidemics

Aside from the countries already discussed – countries with the worst epidemics in 1988, and countries in Southern Africa with the worst epidemics in 2007 – generalized epidemics developed in most if not all other African countries through 2007. In most of these countries, adult HIV prevalence ranged from 1 percent to 4 percent. Through 2005, estimated adult prevalence exceeded 5 percent in only three other countries – Kenya in East Africa, and Cameroon and Gabon in Central Africa.

Kenya is the wealthiest and most developed country in East Africa. Although its HIV epidemic began later than epidemics in Tanzania and Uganda, a 2003 national survey found 6.7 percent of Kenyan adults to be HIV-positive, comparable to HIV prevalence in Tanzania and Uganda. Kenya's epidemic is much worse than what is found in poorer neighbors to the north – Southern Sudan, Ethiopia, and Somalia.

Table 6.4: Distribution of HIV infections in other African countries* with at least 5 percent HIV prevalence in adults

Country, year of survey	HIV prevalence (%) in adults		HIV prevalence (%) in women by education			HIV prevalence (%) in women by wealth quintiles				
	Urban	Rural	None	Prim-ary	Secondary or higher	Low-est	2nd	3rd	4th	High-est
Cameroon, 2004										
Women	8.4	4.8	3.4	7.2	8.2	3.1	4.1	8.1	9.4	8.0
Men	4.9	3.0								
Kenya, 2003										
Women	12.3	7.5	4.4	9.9	8.2	3.9	8.5	7.1	9.7	12.2
Men	7.5	3.6								

*All countries for which survey data are available.
Sources: See the Statistical Annex.

Adult HIV prevalence was likely less than 0.5 percent in Cameroon and somewhat higher in Gabon in the mid-1980s, an estimated 50 years after HIV began to circulate in the region. Some scientists saw 'a paradoxical discrepancy between high genetic diversity,' which was what one would expect to find in an old epidemic, 'and low prevalence.'[30] In both countries, old epidemics expanded in the 1990s. A national survey in Cameroon in 2004 found 5.5 percent of adults to be HIV-positive. For Gabon, UNAIDS estimated 7.9 percent adult HIV prevalence in 2005. Both Cameroon and Gabon are relatively wealthy and developed by African standards, and their HIV prevention programs have cooperated with international advice. Why did their epidemics do so little for so long, and then expand in the 1990s, when prevention programs were in place?

Epidemics in African countries at war

In 1996, UNAIDS stated that 'HIV spreads fastest in conditions of poverty, powerlessness and social instability – conditions that are often at their most extreme during emergencies.'[31] However, evidence shows otherwise. After 1984, when HIV tests have been available to track HIV prevalence, seven African countries have had civil disorders or wars that lasted for a decade or longer. In all seven, HIV epidemics grew slowly or not at all during the war.[32] Moving counterclockwise from West Africa, these countries are Sierra Leone, Liberia, DRC, Angola, Mozambique, Somalia, and Southern Sudan.

Sierra Leone's civil war began in 1991, when rebels from the Revolutionary United Front entered from Liberia. The rebels were notorious for chopping off hands to terrorize the population. For 11 years, the rebels lived off profits from diamond mines. Within months after the war ended in 2002, a survey found that 0.6 percent of adolescents and adults aged 12-49 years had lost a limb during the war, and 6 percent of women reported forced sex by someone other than their regular partner during the past year.[33] The same survey found that only 0.9 percent of adults and adolescents were HIV-positive.

Liberia's civil war began in 1989, when Charles Taylor's National Patriotic Front entered from Cote d'Ivoire. Taylor seized power in 1990. Subsequently, war continued off and on until 2003, when Taylor resigned as president and moved to Nigeria. Surveys before the war found little HIV infection. HIV prevalence increased during the war, but remained low. A national survey in 2006-07 found 1.5 percent adult HIV prevalence.

In DRC, President Mobutu's grip on power slipped with age and with the end of the cold war. In 1991, soldiers rioted to protest low pay, and foreigners fled the breakdown of civil order. In 1996, Laurent Kabila's rebels overthrew Mobutu. Civil war resumed in 1998 with troops from Angola, Rwanda, Uganda, Zimbabwe and other African countries attacking or supporting Kabila's government. After Joseph Kabila replaced his assassinated father in 2001, the central government negotiated and extended its authority over most of the country through mid-2007.

A 1997 study in three cities found that 'HIV seroprevalence rates remain relatively low and stable' despite 'social disruption, the rapid decline in health-care provision, and the decrease in funding in health education programmes.'[34] From the early 1990s to the early 2000s, HIV prevalence fell among women in urban antenatal clinics (see the Statistical Annex). Among mostly rural women from DRC attending antenatal clinics in refugee camps in neighboring countries during 2001-05, HIV prevalence was 1.0-3.4 percent.[35] UNAIDS estimated 3.2 percent adult HIV prevalence in DRC in 2005.

Angola's civil war lasted from independence in 1975 until the death of the rebel leader, Jonas Savimbi, in 2002. In that year, the median HIV prevalence in women attending antenatal clinics in six provinces was 2.4 percent.[36] In 2004, Angola's vice-minister of health noted that 'inland provinces that have been more protected by the effect of war have lower figures of [HIV] prevalence.'[37] Angola's HIV prevalence was significantly lower than in neighboring countries at peace to the south and east.

Civil war in Mozambique lasted from 1976 to 1992. During much of that time, the South African government supported rebels to block Mozambique's aid to South Africa's banned African National Congress. Rebel attacks 'destroyed, looted, or forced to close' 46 percent of rural clinics and health posts through 1988.[38] Mozambique's HIV prevalence stayed low during the war, but took off when peace was achieved. Among women attending antenatal clinics in Maputo (the capital), HIV prevalence rose from 1.2 percent in 1992, when the war ended, to 5.8 percent in 1996, and then to 21 percent in 2004. Parallel increases occurred throughout the country.

The secession of northern Somalia in 1988 sparked Somalia's civil war. In the north, Somaliland emerged as a new state in 1991, which as of 2007 was not recognized by the world community. In the south, militias overthrew the government in 1991. Fighting among militias, Islamic organizations, and foreign forces continued into 2007. In 2004, an estimated 0.9 percent of women attending antenatal clinics in Somalia were HIV-positive, based on information from selected clinics.[39]

Southern Sudanese have fought for autonomy or secession for decades. The first north-south civil war began in 1956 and lasted until 1972. The second began in 1983 and ended in 2005. Another civil war in Darfur, in western Sudan, continued into 2007. In 2002-03, surveys assisted by the US CDC measured HIV prevalence in parts of Southern Sudan controlled by the rebels. Findings from these surveys – particularly, adult HIV prevalence of 0.4 percent in Rumbek town and

0.7 percent in rural areas of Yei County[40] – give a good indication of low HIV prevalence in the south's overwhelmingly rural population at the end of the war.

Two studies published in 2007 present similar evidence for other African countries with shorter or more limited wars. A study assisted by the UN High Commission on Refugees found that data from Burundi, Rwanda, and north Uganda, as well as from several countries considered in previous paragraphs, 'did not show an increase in prevalence of HIV infection during periods of conflict...'[41] The other study developed an index of armed conflict for 37 African countries during 1991-2000. For 15 countries with no armed conflict, average HIV prevalence in urban women in 2000 (averaging each country's median HIV prevalence in urban sentinel antenatal clinics) was more than twice as high as the average for 22 African countries with armed conflict during the decade.[42]

During wars, UNAIDS recognizes 'a strong likelihood that AIDS control activities, whether undertaken by national governments or NGOs, will have been severely disrupted or have broken down altogether.'[43] Hence, it is noteworthy that HIV prevalence in African countries after long-term wars has been almost uniformly lower than in neighboring countries at peace. Certainly, HIV prevention programs have stopped some transmission (for example, by providing condoms). However, the failure of these programs to consistently outperform the 'no program' situation in countries at war shows that their positive impacts are overwhelmed by other factors.

One proposed explanation for low HIV prevalence after long-term wars is that wars isolate people, reducing their sexual contacts with HIV-positive outsiders. Although wars no doubt reduce sexual contacts with visiting truckers, they very likely increase contacts with visiting soldiers. The net impact on sexual exposures to HIV is not clear. Another possible explanation is that wars slow HIV transmission through unsafe healthcare by closing government, mission, and private clinics. This interpretation fits events in Yambuku, DRC, where closing the mission hospital – which had spread Ebola through contaminated injections – stopped the 1976 Ebola outbreak.

Low-level generalized epidemics in Africa

As of 2005, more than 200 million people – almost a third of Africa's population – lived in countries with less than 2 percent HIV prevalence among adults. In at least five countries – Senegal, Niger, Madagascar, Mauritania, and Somalia – less than 1 percent of adults were HIV-positive. HIV prevalence in some of these countries is comparable to what is found in concentrated epidemics in the Americas and Europe. However, these are generalized, not concentrated epidemics – women are infected as often or more often than men (Table 6.5). For example, Senegal's 2002 national survey found that 0.9 percent of women were infected vs. 0.4 percent of men. As in many other African countries, HIV prevalence among women in Ethiopia, Guinea, and Niger increased with education and wealth.

Table 6.5: Distribution of HIV infections in selected African countries with low-level generalized epidemics

Country, year of survey	HIV prevalence (%) in adults		HIV prevalence (%) in women by education			HIV prevalence (%) in women by wealth quintiles				
	Urban	Rural	None	Primary	Secondary or higher	Lowest	2nd	3rd	4th	Highest
Ethiopia, 2005										
Women	7.7	0.6	1.0	2.5	5.5	0.3	1.0	0.4	0.2	6.1
Men	2.4	0.7								
Guinea, 2005										
Women	3.9	0.9	1.3	2.5	5.1	1.4	0.7	0.6	2.8	3.6
Men	0.6	1.1								
Niger, 2006										
Women	1.5	0.5	0.5	1.5	1.2	0.3	0.5	0.4	0.8	1.2
Men	1.3	0.6								
Senegal, 2005										
Women	0.9	0.8	0.9	1.2	0.4					
Men	0.4	0.5								

Sources: See the Statistical Annex.

In African countries with low HIV prevalence, infections notably do not concentrate in promiscuous adults. Information on sexual behavior and HIV prevalence is available from national surveys for five countries with adult HIV prevalence ranging from 0.7 percent to 2.2 percent (Burkina Faso, Ethiopia, Ghana, Guinea, and Niger). In these five countries, women who reported 0-1 sexual partners in the past year had 96-100 percent of HIV infections in women (see Table 7.1). In

113

the same five countries, men who reported 0-1 sexual partners had 56-91 percent of HIV infections in men. Does sexual transmission of HIV from sex workers to clients to wives drive these low-level generalized epidemics? The evidence does not agree. In the same five countries, 60-77 percent of HIV-positive wives had husbands who were HIV-negative (see Table 7.5).

Even so, non-IDU sex workers often have high HIV prevalence in low-level generalized epidemics. For example, nine sentinel surveys in Ethiopia during 1990-2005 reported 36-74 percent of sex workers to be HIV-positive.[44] In generalized epidemics, women in sex work are on the front lines – they are exposed to both blood and sex risks. From available evidence, no one can show what proportions of their HIV infections come from which risks.

Low-level generalized epidemics in the Caribbean

Outside of Africa, the oldest generalized epidemics were recognized in Haiti and in other small countries in the Caribbean region from the 1980s. Currently 10 small countries in the region (Bahamas, Barbados, Belize, Dominican Republic, Haiti, Honduras, Guyana, Jamaica, Suriname, and Trinidad and Tobago) have low-level generalized epidemics, with estimated adult HIV prevalence ranging from 1 percent to 3.3 percent (in the Bahamas). After UNAIDS's 2002 estimate put Haiti's adult HIV prevalence as high as 6.1 percent, a national survey in 2005-06 found only 2.2 percent of adults to be HIV-positive. Taken together, these 10 countries have several hundred thousand HIV infections, less than 1 percent of the world total.

Comparable or higher HIV prevalence in women vs. men shows these are generalized, not concentrated, epidemics. In contrast to Africa, HIV prevalence is almost equal in urban and rural adults in Haiti and the Dominican Republic, and neither socioeconomic status nor education increase risk among Haitian women (Table 6.6). As in other generalized epidemics in Africa, sex workers are at high risk. For example, in Guyana, four sentinel surveys during 1990-00 reported 25-45 percent HIV prevalence in sex workers.[45]

Generalized epidemics in 10 small countries in the Caribbean are growing slowly, if at all. Other regional countries have concentrated epidemics, or possibly mixed epidemics, with low HIV prevalence. In Guatemala and Panama, for example, surveys among women attending antenatal clinics seldom find more than 1 percent to be HIV-positive, and surveys among sex workers seldom find more than 10 percent to be HIV-positive.[46]

Table 6.6: Distribution of HIV infections in Asian and Caribbean countries* with low-level generalized epidemics

Country, year of survey	HIV prevalence (%) in adults		HIV prevalence (%) in women by education			HIV prevalence (%) in women by wealth quintiles				
	Urban	Rural	None	Prim-ary	Secondary or higher	Low-est	2nd	3rd	4th	High-est
Cambodia, 2005										
Women	1.3	0.5	0.8	0.6	0.5	0.5	0.4	0.4	0.8	0.9
Men	1.6	0.4								
Dominican Republic, 2002										
Women	0.9	1.0								
Men	1.0	1.3								
Haiti, 2005-06										
Women	2.7	2.0	2.3	2.6	2.1	2.4	0.9	2.4	3.7	1.9
Men	1.8	2.1								
India, 2005-06										
Women	0.29	0.18	0.27	0.31†	0.10	0.18	0.20	0.24	0.34	0.12
Men	0.41	0.32								

*All countries for which data are available from national surveys.

† From any to not more than 7 years of education.

Sources: See the Statistical Annex.

Low-level generalized epidemics in Asia

Outside Africa and the Caribbean, low-level generalized or mixed epidemics, with estimated adult HIV prevalence ranging from 0.36 percent to 1.8 percent, are found in five countries: Cambodia, India, Myanmar, and Thailand in Asia; and Papua New Guinea in Oceania. These five countries collectively account for 3.5 million of the estimated 27 million increase in global HIV infections from 1988 to 2007. In some other countries with very low HIV prevalence, such as Nepal, information is too limited to reliably characterize their epidemics as concentrated or very low-level mixed or generalized epidemics.

India

After the discovery of HIV in India in 1986, HIV spread rapidly. By 1990, expanded testing found 13-55 percent HIV prevalence in seven

115

sites spanning thousands of kilometers, including sites testing sex workers, IDUs, and people seeking treatment for sexually transmitted diseases.[47] India's National AIDS Control Organization estimated 200,000 HIV infections in 1990, increasing to 3.5 million in 1998.[48] In 2005, UNAIDS estimated that India had 5.7 million infections – more than any other country in the world. However, estimates for 1998 and 2005 were too high.[49] A 2005-06 national survey found 0.28 percent HIV prevalence in adults.[50] Based on the survey, but with some adjustments, the government of India and UNAIDS agreed on an estimate of 0.36 percent adult HIV prevalence and 2.5 million infections in 2006.[51]

The HIV epidemic varies regionally across India, a large country, with a population greater than all of sub-Saharan Africa. Most HIV infections are found in four southern states with a fourth of India's population – Andhra Pradesh, Karnataka, Maharashtra, and Tamil Nadu. In these states, adult HIV prevalence in the 2005-06 survey ranged from 0.34-0.96 percent. In three eastern states with 0.5 percent of India's population – Mizoram, Manipur, and Nagaland – HIV prevalence is also relatively high, due in part to IDUs injecting heroin from Myanmar. The 2005-06 survey found 1.1 percent adult HIV prevalence in Manipur. Other states, with collectively three-quarters of India's population, have an adult HIV prevalence of only 0.12 percent.

Overall, India appears to have a low-level mixed epidemic, with some states having more concentrated or more generalized epidemics. An estimated 1.6 men are infected for every woman, a sex ratio that is intermediate between concentrated and generalized epidemics. Among women, education beyond the primary level reduces risk. On the other hand, greater wealth appears to increase risk among women, except that the highest wealth quintile has lower HIV prevalence (see Table 6.6).

Many AIDS experts have proposed that (heterosexual) sex work accounts for most infections in India, as sex workers infect men who infect wives. A World Bank model showing sex workers driving India's HIV epidemic assumed that 15 percent of men visited sex workers an average of 50 times per year.[52] Overwhelming evidence shows much more conservative sexual behavior.[53] Moreover, in the 2005-06 survey, 39 percent of married, HIV-positive women had HIV-negative husbands (see Chapter 7). Commercial sex no doubt contributes to India's HIV epidemic – but how much does it contribute?

116

Thailand

In 1987-88, the HIV epidemic exploded among IDUs in Bangkok. In the next year, it exploded among (non-IDU) women in sex work in the far north. From 1988 to 1989, HIV prevalence among brothel-based sex workers in Chiang Mai city in north Thailand increased from 0.4 percent to 44 percent.[54] Two studies among sex workers in northern Thailand during 1989-93 show 3.6-17 percent contracting HIV each month (after setting aside those who were already infected).[55] These are among the highest rates of HIV incidence ever observed in any population. Because studies ignored medical injections and other blood exposures, no one knows how much blood exposures contributed to these extraordinarily high rates of HIV incidence.

Unlike Africa, where HIV hit hardest among well-off people in capital cities, Thailand's epidemic was most intense in rural areas of remote provinces in the far north and in other border and coastal provinces. HIV prevalence among Thai army recruits from several districts in the far north approached 20 percent during 1991-93, compared to 2.0-4.0 percent for other regions.[56] In the mid-1990s, HIV prevalence in pregnant women attending antenatal care peaked over 2 percent for the nation.

From these peaks, Thailand's HIV prevalence fell dramatically by 2003 to 0.5 percent in army recruits and just over 1 percent in pregnant women.[57] Because studies continued to ignore blood exposures, there is no basis to allocate credit for reduced HIV transmission across multiple changes, including more condom use and safer healthcare. Currently, Thailand appears to have a mixed epidemic, with an estimated 1.5 men infected for every woman, and MSMs and IDUs accounting for substantial numbers of infections.

Cambodia, Myanmar, and Papua New Guinea

The Paris Peace Agreement in 1991 ended decades of war in Cambodia and led to an influx of aid. Somehow, changes that came with peace appear to have ignited Cambodia's HIV epidemic. At the end of the war in 1991, HIV prevalence in blood donors in Cambodia was only 0.1 percent. During the late 1990s, many surveys among sex workers (especially brothel-based sex workers), police, military personnel, and patients seeking treatment for sexually transmitted

117

disease reported HIV prevalence over 5 percent.[58] A national survey in 2005 found 0.6 percent HIV prevalence among both men and women, describing a low-level generalized epidemic. Among women, HIV prevalence increased with wealth, but decreased with education (see Table 6.6).

IDUs led the expansion of Myanmar's HIV epidemic in the early 1990s, with later spread among sex workers and others. From the late 1990s, almost 2 percent of army recruits have been HIV-positive, and comparable rates of HIV prevalence have been found in pregnant women. These rates stabilized after 2000. In 2005, UNAIDS estimated 1.3 percent of adults to be HIV-positive. As of early 2007, a UN website attributed 30 percent of new HIV infections to IDU,[59] which describes a mixed epidemic.

In Papua New Guinea in Oceania, HIV prevalence among pregnant women attending selected urban antenatal clinics passed 1 percent in 2003-04. UNAIDS estimated adult HIV prevalence at 1.8 percent in 2005 (see the Statistical Annex). As of 2007, there is no indication that the expansion of Papua New Guinea's epidemic has been curbed.

Poverty and generalized HIV epidemics

Many people who write about international health and development link HIV with poverty. A 2002 article in the *American Journal of Public Health* generalized that 'In all societies, regardless of their degree of development or prosperity, the HIV/AIDS epidemic...now affects almost exclusively the most marginalized sectors of society...'[60] A 2004 essay in *Lancet* declared that 'poverty reduction will undoubtedly be at the core of a sustainable solution to HIV/AIDS.'[61]

In a recent book, Eileen Stillwagon presents evidence that malnutrition and diseases linked to poverty – such as malaria, tuberculosis, and parasite infections – increase people's susceptibility to HIV infection, and facilitate HIV transmission from those who are already infected to others.[62] For example, people infected with schistosomiasis, a parasite from snails, often have genital sores that increase risks to acquire and to transmit HIV infection.

Poverty may well impact sexual behavior and biological susceptibility in ways that at times favor HIV transmission. However, national surveys as well as other studies[63] show that people with more wealth are often more likely to be HIV-positive in Africa and also in some Asian countries. Apparently, whatever effects poor nutrition and poverty-related diseases might have to favor HIV transmission, these effects are often overwhelmed by other factors.

The exposures that lead to generalized epidemics appear to vary according to political boundaries. None of the world's richest and most developed countries has a generalized epidemic. But many of the poorest countries similarly do not have generalized epidemics. For adults who are neither MSMs nor IDUs, high risk to acquire HIV infection is not explained by poverty, but appears to be linked in some other way to living in specific countries in Asia, the Caribbean, and especially Africa.

Failure of HIV prevention in countries with generalized epidemics

From 1988 through 2007, the estimated number of HIV infections in countries with generalized epidemics increased from 2.5 million to 25 million. This increase occurred in the face of well-funded HIV prevention programs.

Because HIV prevention programs to date have not consistently stopped generalized epidemics, it is clear that standard programs come with no guarantees for success. There is thus a risk that new generalized epidemics might emerge. Which countries are at risk? Some expert predictions have been far off the mark. For example, in 2002 a US Intelligence Community Assessment predicted 50-75 million HIV infections in China, India, Ethiopia, Russia, and Nigeria by 2010.[64] As of 2007, approximately 7 million people were infected in these five countries, generalized epidemics had not emerged in China or Russia, and low-level epidemics continued in Ethiopia and India.

Probably the best basis for prediction is simply to extrapolate from what has happened to date. For example, in Bangladesh and Indonesia, HIV infections have been observed among IDUs for years without spreading into the general population. In such countries, the conditions – whatever they are – may not support HIV transmission among the general population. On the other hand, African wars appear to suppress generalized epidemics, while Mozambique's epidemic take-off coincided with the end of its civil war in 1992. Thus, African countries with peace after many years of war – such as Angola, Liberia, Sierra Leone, and Southern Sudan – may be the most likely venues for new and fierce generalized epidemics. But without knowing the factors that allow HIV to spread through the general population, such 'blind' extrapolations provide unreliable projections – and no guidance for how to prevent or to restrain generalized epidemics.

---

[1] Table 6.1, estimates of HIV infections in 1988 are from: Sato PA, Chin J, Mann JM. 'Review of AIDS and HIV infection: Global epidemiology and statistics', *AIDS*, 1989, 3 (suppl 1): S301-7; Chin J, Sato PA, Mann JM. 'Projections of HIV infections and AIDS cases to the year 2000', *Bull WHO*, 1990, 68: 1-11.

[2] Table 6.1, estimates of HIV infections in 2007 are from: UNAIDS. *AIDS epidemic update December 2007.* Geneva: UNAIDS, 2007. Table 6.1 includes Sudan in sub-Saharan Africa; includes Belize, Guyana, Honduras, and Suriname as countries with generalized epidemics in the Caribbean region; and includes information on HIV prevalence from recent national surveys (see the Statistical Annex in this book).

[3] CDC. *HIV/AIDS Surveillance Report, 2005*, vol. 17, rev. ed. Atlanta: CDC, 2007; Health Canada. *HIV and AIDS in Canada: Surveillance report to June 30, 2005.* Ottawa: Health Canada, 2005; National Centre in HIV Epidemiology and Clinical Research. *HIV/AIDS, Viral Hepatitis and Sexually Transmissible Infections in Australia: Annual Surveillance Report 2006.* Sydney: National Centre in HIV Epidemiology and Clinical Research, 2006; European Centre for the Epidemiological Monitoring of AIDS. *HIV/AIDS Surveillance in Europe, end-year report 2005*, no. 73. Saint-Maurice, France: EuroHIV, 2005.

[4] Pinkerton SD, Abramson PR, Kalichman SC, et al. 'Secondary HIV transmission rates in a mixed-gender sample', *Int J STD AIDS*, 2000, 11: 38-44.

[5] Aavitsland P, Nilsen O, Lystad AA. 'No evidence of an epidemic of locally acquired heterosexual HIV infection in Norway', *Sex Transm Dis*, 2002, 29: 222-7.

[6] UNAIDS. *2006 Report on the global AIDS epidemic.* Geneva: UNAIDS, 2006.

[7] Twigg JL, Skolnik R. *Evaluation of the World Bank's assistance in responding to the AIDS epidemic: Russia case study.* Washington DC: World Bank, 2005.

[8] European Centre for the Epidemiological Monitoring of AIDS. *HIV/AIDS Surveillance in Europe, mid-year report 2006*, no. 74. Saint-Maurice, France: EuroHIV, 2006.

[9] Zhang K-L, Ma S-J. 'Epidemiology of HIV in China', *BMJ*, 2002, 324: 803-4.

[10] Ministry of Health, China, UNAIDS, WHO. *2005 Update on the HIV/AIDS epidemic and response in China.* Geneva: WHO, 2006.

[11] Quan VM, Chung A, Long HT, et al. 'HIV in Vietnam: The evolving epidemic and the prevention response, 1996 through 1999', *J Acquir Immune Defic Syndr*, 2000, 25: 360-9.

[12] Riono P, Jazant S. 'The current situation of the HIV/AIDS epidemic in Indonesia', *AIDS Educ Prev*, 2004, 16 (suppl A), 78-90.

[13] Pisani E, Lazzari S, Walker N, et al. 'HIV surveillance: A global perspective', *J Acquir Immune Defic Syndr*, 2001, 32 (suppl 1): S3-11.

[14] ORC MACRO. *Ethiopia Demographic and Health Survey 2005*. Calverton, Maryland: ORC MACRO, 2006.

[15] Kwesigabo G, Killewo J, Urassa W, et al. 'HIV-1 infection prevalence and incidence trends in areas of contrasting levels of infection in the Kagera Region, Tanzania, 1987-2000', *J Acquir Immune Defic Syndr*, 2005, 40: 585-91.

[16] Stoneburner RL, Low-Beer D. 'Population-level HIV declines and behavioral risk avoidance in Uganda', *Science*, 2004, 304: 714-18. p. 714.

[17] UNAIDS, WHO. *Uganda: Epidemiological Fact Sheets on HIV/AIDS and Sexually Transmitted Infections, 2002 update*. Geneva: WHO, 2002.

[18] Whitworth JAG, Mahe C, Mbulaiteye SM, et al. 'HIV-1 epidemic trends in rural south-west Uganda over a 10-year period', *Trop Med Inter Health*, 2002, 7: 1047-52.

[19] Allen T. 'AIDS and evidence: Interrogating some Ugandan myths', *J biosoc Sci*, 2006, 38: 7-28. p. 11.

[20] World Bank. *African Development Indicators 1998/99*. Washington DC: World Bank, 1998.

[21] De la Cruz F, Baretto J, Palma de Souza C, et al. 'Seroepidemiological study on HIV-1 and HIV-2 prevalence in Mozambican population [abstract]', *4th Int Conf AIDS*, Stockholm 13-14 June 1988, Abstract 5056.

[22] Shoub BD, Lyons SF, McGillivray GM, et al. 'Absence of HIV infection in prostitutes and women attending sexually-transmitted disease clinics in South Africa', *Trans R Soc Trop Med Hygiene*, 1987, 81: 874-5.

[23] Prior CRB, Buckle GC. 'Blood donors with antibody to the human immunodeficiency virus – the Natal experience', *S Afr Med J*, 1990, 77: 623-5.

[24] US Census Bureau. *HIV/AIDS Surveillance Data Base, June 2003 release*. Washington, DC: US Census Bureau, 2003.

[25] World Bank. *Staff Appraisal Report: Botswana Family Health Project*. Report No. 4820-BT. Washington, DC: World Bank, 1984. p. 6.

[26] World Bank. *African Development Indicators 1998/99*.

[27] 'Botswana President Receives 2001 Harvard AIDS Institute Leadership Award', *Update*, 2002; 3(1): p. 1. Available at: http://www.aids.harvard.edu/news_publications/update/vol3iss1/update3.htm l (accessed 11 September).

[28] Whiteside A, Hickey A, Ngcobo N, et al. *What is driving the HIV/AIDS epidemic in Swaziland, and what more can we do about it?* Mbabane: National Emergency Response Committee on HIV/AIDS, 2003. p. 6.

[29] Heywood M. 'The price of denial', *Development Update* 2005; 5: 93-122. Available at: http://www.alp.org.za/modules.php?op=modload&name=News&file=article&s id=236 (accessed 5 November 2007).

[30] Makuwa M, Souquiere S, Apetrei C, et al. 'HIV prevalence and strain diversity in Gabon: the end of a paradox [letter]', *AIDS*, 2000, 14: 1275.

[31] UNAIDS. *Guidelines for HIV Interventions in Emergency Settings*. Geneva: WHO, 1996. p. 2.

[32] Gisselquist D. 'Impact of long-term civil disorders and wars on the trajectory of HIV epidemics in sub-Saharan Africa', *J Soc Aspects HIV/AIDS*, 2004, 1: 114-27.

[33] Kaiser R, Spiegel P, Salama P, et al. *HIV/AIDS seroprevalence and behavioral risk factor survey in Sierra Leone, April 2002*. Atlanta: CDC, no date.

[34] Mulanga-Kabeya C, Nzilambi N, Edidi B, et al. 'Evidence of stable HIV seroprevalence in selected populations in the Democratic Republic of the Congo', *AIDS*, 1998, 12: 905-10. p. 908.

[35] Spiegel PB, Bennedsen AR, Claass J, et al. 'Prevalence of HIV infection in conflict-affected and displaced people in seven sub-Saharan African countries: A systematic review', *Lancet*, 2007, 369: 2187-95.

[36] WHO, Regional Office for Africa (WHO/AFRO). *HIV/AIDS Epidemiological Surveillance Update for the WHO Africa Region*. Zimbabwe: WHO/AFRO, 2003.

[37] Health Systems Trust. 'Angola: HIV infection rate for pregnant women at 2.8%.', Health Systems Trust, 2004. Available at: http://www.hst.org.za/news/20040592 (accessed 9 September 2007).

[38] Finnegan W. *A Complicated War: The harrowing of Mozambique*. Berkeley: University of California Press, 1992. p. 24.

[39] Spiegel PB et al. 'Prevalence of HIV infection'.

[40] Kaiser R, Kedamo T, Lane J, et al. 'HIV, syphilis, herpes simplex virus 2, and behavioral surveillance among conflict-affected populations in Yei and Rumbek, southern Sudan', *AIDS*, 2006, 20: 942-4.

[41] Spiegel PB et al. 'Prevalence of HIV infection'. p. 2187.

[42] Strand RT, Dias LF, Bergstrom S, et al. 'Unexpected low prevalence of HIV among fertile women in Luanda, Angola. Does war prevent the spread of HIV?', *Int J STD AIDS*, 2007, 18: 467-71.

[43] UNAIDS. *Guidelines for HIV interventions in emergency settings*. p. 2.

[44] UNAIDS, WHO. *Ethiopia: Epidemiological Fact Sheets on HIV/AIDS and Sexually Transmitted Infections, December 2006*. Geneva: WHO, 2006.

[45] UNAIDS, WHO. *Guyana: Epidemiological Fact Sheets on HIV/AIDS and Sexually Transmitted Infections, December 2006*. Geneva: WHO, 2006.

[46] UNAIDS, WHO. *Guatemala: Epidemiological Fact Sheets on HIV/AIDS and Sexually Transmitted Infections, December 2006*. Geneva: WHO, 2006; UNAIDS, WHO. *Panama: Epidemiological Fact Sheets on HIV/AIDS and Sexually Transmitted Infections, December 2006*. Geneva: WHO, 2006.

[47] UNAIDS, WHO. *India: Epidemiological Fact Sheets on HIV/AIDS and Sexually Transmitted Infections, 2004 update*. Geneva: WHO, 2004.

[48] National AIDS Control Organization (NACO). 'An overview of the spread and prevalence of HIV/AIDS in India'. Available at: http://nacoonline.org/facts_overview.htm (accessed 9 September 2007).

[49] Dandona L, Lakshmi V, Sudha T, et al. 'A population-based study of human immunodeficiency virus in south India reveals major differences from sentinel surveillance-based estimates', *BMC Med*, 2006, 4: 31.

[50] International Institute for Population Sciences (IIPS), ORC Macro. *National Family Health Survey (NFHS-3), 2005-06: India: Vol. 1*. Mumbai: IIPS, 2006. Available at: http://www.nfhsindia.org/volume_1.html (accessed 18 October 2007).

[51] Kalyan R. 'AIDS cases: Dharwad tops list', *Deccan Herald*, 7 July 2007.

[52] Over M, Heywood P, Gold J, et al. *HIV/AIDS Treatment and Prevention in India: Modeling the cost and consequences*. Washington DC: World Bank, 2004. p. 65.

[53] Gisselquist D, Correa M. 'How much does heterosexual commercial sex contribute to India's HIV epidemic?', *Int J STD AIDS*, 2006, 17: 736-42.

[54] Siraprapasiri T, Thanprasertsuk S, Rodklay A, et al. 'Risk factors for HIV among prostitutes in Chiangmai, Thailand', *AIDS*, 1991; 5: 579-82.

[55] Sawanpanyalert P, Ungchusak K, Thanprasertsuk S, et al. 'HIV-1 seroconversion rates among female commercial sex workers, Chiang Mai, Thailand: A multi cross-sectional study', *AIDS*, 1994; 8: 825-9; Gray JA, Dore GJ, Li Y, et al. 'HIV-1 infection among female commercial sex workers in rural Thailand', *AIDS*, 1997; 11: 89-94.

[56] Sirisopana N, Torugsa K, Mason CJ, et al. 'Correlates of HIV-1 sereopositivity among young men in Thailand', *J Acquir Immune Defic Syndr*, 1996, 11: 492-8.

[57] Punpanich W, Ungchusak K, Detels R. 'Thailand's response to the HIV epidemic: Yesterday, today, and tomorrow', *AIDS Educ Prev*, 2004, 16 (suppl A): 119-36.

[58] US Census Bureau. *HIV/AIDS Surveillance Data Base, June 2003 release*.

[59] UNDP. 'Youandaids: The HIV/AIDS portal for Asia.' Available at: http://www.youandaids.org/Asia%20Pacific%20at%20a%20Glance/Myanmar/index.asp (accessed 9 September 2007).

[60] Parker R. 'The global HIV/AIDS pandemic, structural inequalities, and the politics of international health', *Am J Pub Health*, 2002, 92: 343-6. p. 344.

[61] Fenton L. 'Preventing HIV/AIDS through poverty reduction: The only sustainable solution?' *Lancet*, 2004, 364: 1186-7. pp. 1186-7.

[62] Stillwagon E. *AIDS and the Ecology of Poverty*. Oxford: Oxford University Press, 2006.

[63] Wojcicki JM. 'Socioeconomic status as a risk factor for HIV infection in women in East Central, and Southern Africa: A systematic review', *J biosoc Sci*, 2005, 37: 1-36.

[64] National Intelligence Council. 'The next wave of HIV/AIDS: Nigeria, Ethiopia, Russia, India, and China.' Available at: http://www.dni.gov/nic/special_nextwaveHIV.html (accessed 9 September 2007).

Chapter 7

NOT LISTENING, AND NOT EXPLAINING THE EPIDEMIC, 1989-2007

> Informed opinion and active co-operation on the part of the public are of the utmost importance in the improvement of the health of the people.
>
> – Constitution of the World Health Organization, 1946[1]

One-way communication from health experts to the public has characterized and damaged the response to HIV in countries with generalized epidemics. Researchers have not worked with HIV-positive adults to trace the source of their infections, and health experts have not believed HIV-positive adults who deny heterosexual risks.

From racial stereotypes to stigma

From racial stereotypes to hypothesis

Through the early 1990s, most AIDS experts supposed that the spread of HIV among the general population in Africa, but not in the US or Europe, was largely due to Africans having more sexual partners than Americans or Europeans. Stillwagon attributes misunderstanding of Africa's AIDS epidemic to 'Centuries-old stereotypes that emphasize exotic and exceptional sexuality' in Africa.[2] In 1989, one journal article described Africans as susceptible to AIDS because they are less cautious, more impulsive, less inhibited sexually, and less intelligent.[3] This unusually crude presentation resonated with widely held views of African sexual behavior.

In 1991, Packard and Epstein criticized the 'premature closure of African AIDS research.'[4]

> ...[A]ssumptions about the importance of sexual promiscuity in the transmission of HIV in Africa were initially based on limited, and in some cases methodologically questionable data. These assumptions, nonetheless, served to shape both the questions which AIDS researchers asked and the way in which they interpreted data. This

narrowing of research in turn discouraged serious consideration of the role of alternative avenues of transmission…

We are in fact much further from understanding the epidemiology of AIDS in Africa than some medical researchers, development officers, and social scientists would have us believe…

As early as 1989-90, surveys of sexual behavior coordinated by the Global Programme on AIDS in 12 African countries challenged stereotypes of African sexual behavior. Evidence from these surveys was 'totally incompatible with the view…that the HIV pandemic in Africa was fueled by extreme promiscuity…The results from the African surveys do not portray a region with uniquely high levels of partner change.'[5] Furthermore, these surveys showed big differences in sexual behavior from one African country to another – differences that did not correspond to differences in HIV prevalence.

In national surveys in 14 African countries and Haiti during 2003-06, over 90 percent of women reported 0-1 sexual partners in the past year, and these women accounted for 89 percent to 100 percent of HIV infections in women (Table 7.1). Across the same 15 countries, men who reported 0-1 sexual partners in the past year accounted for 48 percent to 97 percent of HIV infections in men. Similarly, surveys in Cambodia and India found little or no concentration of HIV infections in the small minority of adults reporting two or more sexual partners in the past year.

In 2006, a prominent review of information on sexual behavior around the world reported a 'comparatively high prevalence of multiple partnerships in developed countries, compared with parts of the world with far higher rates of sexually transmitted infections and HIV, such as African countries…'[6]

Nevertheless, some experts have continued to argue that distinctive patterns of heterosexual behavior have been responsible for Africa's ferocious AIDS epidemics. In recent years, the most common formulation of this argument has been that Africans have more concurrent partners (more than one ongoing relationship). For example, a book published in 2007, relying on data selected from surveys in several countries during 1989-90, generalized that 'From 20% to 40% of sexually active adults (both males and females) in many SSA [sub-Saharan African] populations' have 'unprotected sex with multiple and concurrent sex partners.'[7] Clearly, diverse views of

African sexual behavior have survived findings from years of research, and continue to influence experts' explanations of Africa's HIV epidemics.

Table 7.1: Proportions of men and women aged 15-49 years reporting 0-1 sexual partners in the past year, and proportions of HIV infections in such men and women, in 17 countries with generalized epidemics*

Country, year of survey	Adult HIV preva-lence (%)	Women reporting 0-1 sex partners last year		Men reporting 0-1 sex partners last year	
		% of all women	% of HIV-positive women	% of all men	% of HIV-positive men
Africa					
Ethiopia, 2005	1.6	100	99	98	<90
Rwanda, 2005	3.0	100	99	97	97
Zimbabwe, 2005-06	18.1	99	98	91	90
Malawi, 2004	11.8	99	98	90	85
Ghana, 2003	2.2	99	97	90	89
Niger, 2006	0.7	99	100	88	70
Burkina Faso, 2003	1.8	99	97	85	91
Kenya, 2003	6.7	98	95	89	78
Uganda, 2004-05	6.4	97	95	79	66
Guinea. 2005	1.5	97	96	75	56
Cote d'Ivoire, 2005	4.7	96	93	75	75
Tanzania, 2003	7.0	95	93	79	78
Cameroon, 2004	5.5	95	91	70	48
Lesotho, 2004	23.5	92	89	77	70
Asia and the Caribbean					
India, 2005-06	0.28	100	99	99	97
Cambodia, 2005	0.6	100	100	94	79
Haiti, 2005-06	2.2	99	94	77	76

* All countries for which data are available from national surveys.
Note: Percentages of women and of HIV-positive women with 0-1 sex partners are calculated from published data from national surveys by subtracting the number of women and of HIV-positive women with two or more sex partners from totals for women. Percentages for men are calculated in the same way.
Sources: See the Statistical Annex.

From hypothesis to stigma

In 1987, Jonathan Mann distinguished three epidemics related to HIV. The first was the spread of HIV infection. The second was the spread of AIDS disease in persons infected with HIV. The third epidemic was the 'denial, blame, stigmatization, prejudice and discrimination which the fear of AIDS brings out in individuals and societies.'[8]

In Africa and later in other countries with generalized epidemics, HIV prevention messages that attributed almost all HIV infections in adults to heterosexual exposures – messages which grew out of the hypothesis that African promiscuity caused generalized epidemics – spread this third epidemic. Such messages 'educated' the public to see HIV infection as a sign – stigma – of sexual promiscuity. In effect, these HIV prevention messages translated racial stereotypes of sexual behavior into stigma against HIV-positive men and women. Of course, people must be warned about sexual risks – the problem was the lack of attention to other risks, including especially risks in 'virtuous' behaviors such as seeking healthcare or dental care.

In *The Scarlet Letter*, an early American novel, Hester Prynne becomes pregnant by someone other than her absent husband. The community forces her to go around wearing a large red 'A' to mark her as an adultress. Unlike pregnancy, an HIV infection is not a reliable sign of sexual activity. But that is not the impression people in generalized epidemics have got from HIV prevention messages.

Discrimination against HIV-positive people is due in part to mistaken fears that the disease may spread through casual contact – such as sharing eating utensils – and in part to aversion to serious illness from any cause. But an important contributor to discrimination is the belief that almost all HIV infections in adults in countries with generalized epidemics come from sex. Many organizations have tried to fight stigma by encouraging people not to be so critical of promiscuous behavior – which is both controversial and difficult.

Another way to defuse stigma is to spread the message that an HIV infection is not a reliable sign of sexual exposure to HIV. Some AIDS experts have obstructed such messages, arguing that public discussion of iatrogenic transmission will 'detract from prevention efforts aimed at reducing the sexual transmission of HIV'[9] and lead to 'behavioral disinhibition.'[10] These arguments reflect negative perceptions of peoples' intelligence and sexual behavior – that they cannot understand risks, and that they will use any excuse to be sexually promiscuous without condoms. For health experts, these arguments are also a self-serving excuse not to acknowledge nosocomial infections, and thereby to violate medical ethics by not warning people about risks in health care (see Chapters 9 and 10).

Stigma and limited testing obstruct public knowledge of the epidemic

Until well into the 1990s, the AIDS epidemic was invisible to most Africans. In the late 1980s, less than 1 percent of adults were HIV-positive in most communities. Thus, even in communities where HIV prevalence soared over 10 percent in the 1990s, annual deaths from AIDS often did not reach 1 in 100 adults until the late 1990s. Besides, many AIDS-related deaths could be attributed to other causes.

During the 1990s, testing was not a priority in international AIDS programs. When an article in *Lancet* proposed home-based testing to make it easier for people in developing countries to learn their HIV status,[11] WHO's experts objected, arguing that there was no evidence telling people their HIV status would reduce transmission, and that no care was available, so 'the only promise offered here is the potential rejection of the HIV-positive person.'[12] Several World Bank experts whom I spoke with around 2000 worried that telling unmarried African men their HIV status might increase sexual transmission of HIV, because men who learned they were infected might stop using condoms and sleep with as many women as possible.

During the 1990s, getting an HIV test was onerous and/or expensive for most Africans. In a review of HIV testing services in 21 African countries in 2001, only seven countries reported more than 20 government testing sites, and only five reported any testing in the private sector.[13] As of 2000, Piot, the executive director of UNAIDS, estimated that only 5 percent of HIV-positive people in developing countries were aware of their infection, and judged that 'In Africa there is basically only one country where access to testing and counselling is reasonable, and that is Uganda.'[14]

For people in generalized epidemics, the best information they had during the 1990s that HIV was spreading through their communities were reports from sentinel surveys that tested pregnant women in antenatal clinics. But because these surveys disconnected blood samples from names before testing for HIV, no one knew who was infected. Thus, even as governments reported HIV prevalence soaring among women at antenatal clinics, people looked at their own and their spouses' sexual behavior, and supposed that others – sex workers, clients, bad people – were the ones who were infected. For example, in a 2000-01 study among Zambian women who did not know their HIV status, more than half the women who were HIV-positive considered themselves to be at no or low risk for HIV infection.[15]

The belief that sexual exposures accounted for most HIV infections and the stigma that linked HIV to sexual misbehavior were mutually reinforcing. People who had no sexual risks were unlikely to seek HIV tests. Most people who found themselves to be HIV-positive – with or without sexual risks – tried to hide their infections. However, people with recognized sexual risks, such as sex workers and widows of men who had died from AIDS, were less able to do so. Public awareness of AIDS in people with recognized sexual risks supported the view that all HIV came from sex.

Even for counselors and doctors who saw and interviewed HIV-positive people, the belief that HIV infection in adults was a sign of sexual behavior often limited what they could see. For example, doctors and counselors interviewed during a study in India in 2005 explained, 'Men are like that, they go out and then come home and infect their wives; how can we believe when they tell us that they have not had sex outside marriage?' and 'He is a truck driver, what can you expect?'[16]

Because so few people knew they were infected, and because stigma discouraged even those few from talking about their condition, the public knew very little about what was happening from personal experience. Even after tens of millions had been infected, and millions had died, the public's ideas about the presence of AIDS in their communities, and of how HIV was spreading, depended almost entirely on what public health authorities told them. In this situation, if health authorities did not, either deliberately or inadvertently, provide full and accurate information, what people believed about risks for HIV infection could wander far from reality.

Testing and not telling in AIDS research

Poor communication between AIDS experts and research participants – including the ethically dubious practice of withholding life-saving information – has undermined and blighted HIV research in Africa. From the late 1980s and continuing into the 21st century, prominent research projects funded by foreign governments and institutions have tested and followed HIV-positive and HIV-negative Africans without telling them the results of their HIV tests. In these projects, researchers watched adults who did not know they were HIV-positive infect unsuspecting spouses, watched them sicken and die, watched HIV-positive women birth and infect children, and watched the children die.

Testing and not telling not only exposed research participants and their spouses and children to unnecessary risk, but also showed disrespect for the participants' ability to help researchers to identify risks. Researchers who did not tell Africans they were infected were not able to work with them to trace the source of their infections. Thus, testing and not telling not only kept Africans in the dark about their HIV infections, but also kept researchers in the dark about the factors that made Africa's HIV epidemics the worst in the world.

In such projects, researchers have characteristically offered participants a free additional HIV test with counseling at a nearby clinic. Many did not go for this. From this, the researchers' defense for following people who did not know they were HIV-positive has been that they did not want to know.

But there is another way to approach the issue. If someone does not want to receive the results of their HIV test, the researcher can refuse to enroll them in the study. In 1988, the US Office for Protection from Research Risks established a policy that 'Individuals may not be given the option "not to know" the result, either at the time of consenting to be tested or thereafter.'[17] One project that followed that policy in Kigali, Rwanda, from 1988 had no problem enrolling pregnant women in research: '[A]ll but a handful of women wanted to know their test results and many requested that HIV testing and counseling be provided to their spouses as well.'[18]

However, the US policy allowed exceptions. From 1989, researchers funded by the US government began a large study in Rakai, Uganda, testing and enrolling men and women without insisting they learn their HIV status. The study followed and retested thousands of adults, and continued at least into 2006. During 1994-98, the Rakai project followed hundreds of discordant couples. In a large sub-sample of these couples, just over half the HIV-positive partners 'had requested and received HIV counseling, ...25% stated that they had informed their partners,' and 'Condom use was low...'[19] With many participants not knowing that they or their spouses were infected, the project observed 50 incident infections in men and 40 in women with HIV-positive partners.[20]

Similarly, a project in Mwanza, Tanzania, during 1991-94 observed six incident infections in men and women with HIV-positive partners. The study team noted:[21]

> In most prospective studies, intensive counseling of discordant couples has resulted in the adoption of safer sexual practices, and this has limited their capacity to examine risk factors and transmission rates. In the Mwanza study...cohort members were only informed of their HIV status if they accessed a parallel voluntary counseling and testing service. Only a small number of participants pursued this service.

During 1997-2000, the Zimbabwe Vitamin A for Mothers and Babies (ZVITAMBO) study tested and followed over 4,000 HIV-positive women and their newborn children, observing HIV infections and deaths in the children.[22] As the study was designed,[23]

> Mothers could learn their [HIV test] results at any time during the study..., but they were not required to do so. This feature makes ZVITAMBO unique. All other studies of infant feeding and HIV have been conducted among mothers who know their HIV status.

Less than 20 percent of women chose to learn their HIV status. Ninety-two percent of HIV-positive mothers were still breastfeeding at one year.[24] With prolonged breastfeeding, the project observed 64 incident infections in children between the ages of 12 and 24 months. If the project had told women they were HIV-positive and might infect their children, could the women have managed replacement feeding, or at least weaned children after 6 months? These were urban women, in one of the wealthier countries in Africa. More than 80 percent of the women and more than 90 percent of their husbands had received at least 8 years of education.

Table 7.2 lists funders for the three projects discussed in previous paragraphs. Many other research projects in Africa similarly tested and followed adults who did not know they were HIV-positive.

Table 7.2: Funders for selected studies that followed HIV-positive Africans who did not know they were infected

Where and when	Who was followed?	Who paid for the research?
Uganda, Rakai, from 1989 to at least 2006[25]	Adults, including couples, and some infants	National Institute of Allergy and Infectious Diseases, US; National Institute of Child Health and Development, US; Rockefeller Foundation; Fogarty Foundation; GlaxoWellcome Foundation; John Snow Inc.; Pfizer Inc.
Tanzania, Mwanza, 1991-94[26]	Adults, including couples	Commission of the European Communities; Center for International Migration and Development, Germany; Department for International Development, UK; Medical Research Council, UK
Zimbabwe, Harare, 1997-2000[27]	Mothers and infants	Canadian International Development Agency; USAID; Bill and Melinda Gates Foundation; Rockefeller Foundation; BASF (Ludwigshafen, Germany)

Sources: See references by row.

Institutional review boards approved these projects. Even so, these and other similar projects in Africa compare unfavorably to the widely criticized Tuskegee Study of Untreated Syphilis in the Negro Male. From 1932 to 1972, the Tuskegee Study followed African-American men with syphilis, watching them sicken and die without treating their syphilis. The men had tertiary syphilis, so they could not transmit to others, but they suffered heart disease, dementia, and other health damage. Participants in HIV research in Africa who did not know they were HIV-positive not only sickened and died but also passed HIV to spouses and children. Despite the Nuremberg Code,[28] the World Medical Association Declaration of Helsinki,[29] and other documents that provide ethical guidelines for medical research, it is a continuing challenge to recognize and to stop unethical research, particularly in Africa.

Disbelieving people who deny sexual exposures

Another manifestation of researchers and other AIDS experts disrespecting people living with HIV, and what they have to teach others about the epidemic, is the common practice among AIDS experts of disbelieving HIV-positive people who deny sexual exposures to HIV. From the 1980s, substantial numbers of HIV-positive men and women in countries with generalized epidemics have reported never having penetrative sex.

Table 7.3: HIV prevalence in virgin men and women aged 15-49 years in countries with generalized epidemics*

Countries	HIV prevalence (%)			
	All women	Virgin women	All men	Virgin men
Africa				
Burkina Faso, 2003	1.8	0.5	1.9	0.8
Cameroon, 2004	6.8	0.7	4.1	1.0
Cote d'Ivoire, 2005	6.4	0.0	2.9	0.4
Ethiopia, 2005	1.9	0.1	0.9	0.2
Ghana, 2003	2.7	0.0	1.5	0.2
Guinea, 2005	1.9	0.1	0.9	0.6
Kenya, 2003	8.7	1.6	4.6	0.9
Lesotho, 2004	26.4	5.0	19.3	3.7
Malawi, 2004	13.3	2.5	10.2	1.8
Niger, 2006	0.7	0.2	0.7	0.2
Rwanda, 2005	3.6	0.8	2.3	0.2
Tanzania, 2003	7.7	1.4	6.3	2.4
Uganda, 2004-05	7.5	0.8	5.0	0.2
Zimbabwe, 2005-06	21.1	3.9	14.5	2.7
Asia and the Caribbean				
Cambodia, 2005-06	0.6	0.1	0.6	0.0
Haiti, 2005-06	2.3	0.0	2.0	0.2
India, 2005-06	0.22	0.03	0.36	0.13

* All countries for which data are available from national surveys.
Sources: See the Statistical Annex.

In a national survey of women aged 15-19 years in Zimbabwe during 2001-02, 41 percent of 192 women who were HIV-positive reported having no sex partners ever.[30] South Africa's 2005 national survey found 4.3 percent HIV prevalence and (using special blood tests to differentiate new from old infections) a rate of incidence of 1.5 percent per year among adults who reported no sexual partners ever.[31] In national surveys in 17 countries with generalized epidemics during

2003-06, HIV prevalence ranged from 0 percent to 5.0 percent in women who claimed to be virgins, and from 0 percent to 3.7 percent in men who claimed to be virgins (Table 7.3).

In addition, many studies in Africa have found HIV prevalence or incidence in adults who are not virgins, but who report no possible sexual exposures to HIV. For example, a study in Zimbabwe during 1999-2003 followed more than 1,000 initially HIV-negative women. After three years, another round of HIV tests found 48 women with new infections. Twelve of these 48 women reported no sexual partners after their last HIV-negative test. Surprisingly, women reporting no sexual partners acquired HIV faster than women who reported one or more sex partners (1.6 percent vs. 1.2 percent per year).[32] South Africa's 2005 national survey found the same rate of HIV incidence – 2.4 percent per year – in non-virgin adults who reported no sex partners in the past 12 months as in adults who reported one or more sex partners in that period.[33]

Many researchers have routinely interpreted HIV infections in Africans who deny sexual exposures as evidence that they have misreported their sexual behavior.[34] There is no doubt that people often lie and sometimes forget, and it is good science to question evidence. However, it is not good science to reject unwelcome evidence for twenty years without doing what is necessary to collect 'solid' evidence that one trusts to test an hypothesis.

Researchers wear blinders

As described in previous sections, researchers have often not told research participants that they are infected, and so have not been able to work with them to trace the source of their infections. Researchers have also routinely disbelieved research participants who deny sexual exposures, and they have seldom asked about blood exposures. Here are several examples of research designed and implemented in ways that deny and ignore information on risks for HIV infection.

Example of faulty research among African men

During 2002-06, three studies – in South Africa,[35] Uganda,[36] and Kenya[37] – solicited men wanting to be circumcised, then on a random basis circumcised some men first, but told others to wait. Following

135

and retesting circumcised and uncircumcised men, the studies reported that circumcised men acquired HIV infection only 24-45 percent as fast as uncircumcised men. These reported results support the view that circumcision reduces men's risk to acquire HIV from sexual partners. However, because the studies did not investigate or report all risks, it's not clear what happened. Incomplete reports from these trials may mislead men to ignore important risks.

If one believes the men's reported sexual behavior, many of their infections came from non-sexual risks. In the South African trial, 23 (of 69) incident infections occurred in men who reported no unprotected sex during the relevant observation interval (the time from their last negative test to their first positive test). Similarly, in Uganda, 16 (of 67) infections occurred in men who reported no sex partners (6 infections) or 100 percent condom use (10 infections). The trial in Kenya did not report how sexual exposures related to HIV incidence – except for seven men infected in the first three months (sensitive tests did not find HIV in the men's blood at the beginning of the trial). Five of the seven men, including three of four who had been circumcised, reported no sexual exposures from the beginning of the trial until their first HIV-positive test.

None of the studies reported injections or other blood exposures. In the two studies that reported information on genital symptoms, 30-43 percent of incident HIV infections occurred during intervals when men reported genital ulcers or other genital symptoms or problems. Because genital symptoms were more common in uncircumcised men, they may have been more likely to contract HIV infection from skin-piercing tests and treatments, but the studies did not consider that possibility. In the Kenyan trial, circumcision might have infected four men whose infections were recognized one month later, but the study did not mention that possibility. (Notably, in several African countries where men are circumcised during puberty or later, circumcised vs. uncircumcised adolescent men were more likely to be HIV-positive, and this was true both for virgin men and for non-virgins.)[38]

Although two of the three studies (in Kenya and Uganda) told men their HIV status, neither of these studies worked with men with incident infections to see if their sexual partners were the source of their infections. Considering how few partners were involved in the Ugandan study – men reported more than one sexual partner during less than a third of the observation intervals, and 47 percent of the men were married – tracing and testing most of the men's partners, with the men's permission, would appear to have been feasible.

These studies, with their ignored evidence (on sexual exposures) and missing evidence (on blood exposures and on HIV status of sexual partners), launched programs to circumcise millions of African men. These programs may alleviate HIV epidemics, although information on HIV prevalence in circumcised and uncircumcised men from national surveys in 12 African countries (see Table 7.4) suggests otherwise.

If one believes what the men reported about their sexual behavior, a lot of the observed incidence must have come from blood exposures. If so, an alternate or at least complementary strategy to cut HIV incidence may be to improve infection control in hospitals and clinics, including clinics treating sexually transmitted disease. Moreover, if a lot of the incidence was from blood exposures, then programs to circumcise millions of men should be carried out with extreme caution. But because the studies did not ask about or investigate non-sexual risks, the studies cannot guide interventions to address them.

Finally, none of the three trials reported their findings in a way that showed HIV incidence per 1,000 sexual exposures with and without circumcision. This information is important for uncircumcised men. It allows each man to weigh his expected benefits from circumcision – based on his anticipated sexual behavior – against costs and risks. In effect, the study teams simply told African men to get circumcised, rather than fully reporting relevant data to enable men to make their own informed decisions.

Example of faulty research among African women

A study of HIV incidence in pregnant women in Rakai, Uganda,[39] illustrates similar faults. During 1994-99, researchers in Rakai observed much higher HIV incidence in unmarried pregnant women (9.9 percent per year) than in married pregnant women (1.6 percent per year) or in non-pregnant unmarried or married women (1.6 percent and 1.0 percent per year, respectively).

Even though relatively high incidence was strikingly concentrated in unmarried pregnant women, the study proposed that hormonal changes during pregnancy increased women's susceptibility to acquire HIV from sexual partners. Other reported evidence suggested that sexual transmission could not easily explain observed differences in

HIV incidence. Notably, all pregnant women, married and unmarried, who acquired HIV infections reported no sexual partner other than the fetus' father in the past year.

The study did not consider that unmarried pregnant women were more likely to seek abortions than married pregnant women, and to contract HIV during abortions. Ignoring this risk, the study did not report available data on pregnancy loss,[40] which they could have used to test this hypothesis. This alternate hypothesis has obvious implications for HIV prevention. Moreover, the study did not tell women their HIV status, and so did not benefit from their views about how they might have been infected, and did not work with them to trace the source of their infections.

Failing to explain generalized HIV epidemics

Although penile-vaginal coitus transmits HIV between men and women, rates of transmission per coital act and per year are low. From studies of discordant couples in the US, Europe, and Africa, widely quoted estimates of transmission per coital act range from 0.05 percent to 0.11 percent, or once every 900 to 2,000 events.[41] Similarly, most studies of HIV transmission between discordant couples – even when couples are not aware that one partner is HIV-positive – report that not more than 10 percent of the HIV-negative spouses contract HIV from their husbands or wives during a year.[42] With these low rates of transmission, something extraordinary is required to explain how heterosexual coitus could create generalized HIV epidemics, especially the terrible epidemics found in Southern Africa and in many cities in East and Central Africa.

The first idea, that Africans were outrageously promiscuous, fell to evidence in the early 1990s. Over the ensuing fifteen years, a host of other hypotheses supposed that one or more sex-related factors accelerate sexual transmission enough to create generalized epidemics. Although many behaviors or physical conditions are personal risks to acquire or to transmit HIV through sex, studies have been unable to show that these factors explain differences in HIV prevalence between Africa and Europe, or across African countries.

For example, having a genital ulcer is a personal risk – people are more likely to acquire HIV infection from sexual partners if either has a genital ulcer than if neither does. However, studies across Africa have found that communities in which more people have genital ulcers, gonorrhea, herpes simplex virus type 2 (genital herpes), or other sexually transmitted diseases do not consistently have greater HIV prevalence or incidence than communities in which fewer people have these conditions.[43]

Similarly, some experts aver that higher HIV prevalence in Africa is due to Africans having more concurrent (overlapping) sexual partners than people in other continents.[44] Having two ongoing sexual partnerships may be a personal risk to acquire and to transmit HIV. However, African communities in which more people have concurrent partners do not consistently have higher HIV prevalence than other African communities.[45]

From the late 1980s and continuing, some people have argued that lack of male circumcision – which may be a personal risk for men to acquire HIV infection – explains high HIV prevalence in some African communities.[46] A lot of evidence is inconsistent with this hypothesis (see Table 7.4). For example, Rwanda, with only 10 percent of men circumcised, has only 3 percent HIV prevalence in adults, and saw little epidemic growth from 1986 to 2005. Over the same period, adult HIV prevalence in Lesotho, with 59 percent of men circumcised, increased from 0 percent to 24 percent. Although most men in India, China, and Western Europe are uncircumcised, their HIV prevalence – even including MSMs and IDUs – is less than 0.5 percent. Finally, in 7 of 12 African countries with data from national surveys, HIV prevalence was higher in circumcised than in uncircumcised men (see the last three columns on the right in Table 7.4).

Considering the often 100-fold difference between HIV prevalence in non-IDU and non-MSM adults in generalized compared to concentrated epidemics, if sexual factors account for those differences, they should not be so hard to find. Money for research has not been a problem, nor has access to Africans willing to participate in research. From the late 1980s through 2007, researchers looking for the risks that cause Africa's HIV epidemics have followed tens of thousands of HIV-negative Africans for periods ranging from less than a year to more than 15 years, and have observed thousands of incident HIV infections. Even so, researchers have been unable to identify sexual behaviors or conditions which distinguish African countries with the worst HIV epidemics from other African countries or from European countries with concentrated epidemics.

Table 7.4: Percentage of men circumcised, and HIV prevalence in adults and in circumcised and uncircumcised men in countries with generalized epidemics*

Countries, year of survey	% of men circum- cised†	HIV prevalence (%) in			Ratio of HIV prevalence in circumcised vs. uncircumcised men
		Adults aged 15-49 years	Circum- cised ment	Uncircum- cised ment	
Africa					
Rwanda, 2005	10	3.0	3.8	2.7	1.4
Zimbabwe, 2005-06	11	18	20	19	1.1
Malawi, 2004	20‡	12	13‡	9.5‡	1.4
Uganda, 2004-05	26	6.4	4.7	7.4	0.64
Lesotho, 2004	59	24	26	25	1.0
Tanzania, 2003	71	7.0	7.5	7.4	1.0
Kenya, 2003	88	6.7	3.7	21	0.18
Ethiopia, 2005	88	1.6	1.2	1.3	0.93
Burkina Faso, 2003	90	1.8	2.1	4.2	0.50
Cameroon, 2004	93	5.5	5.1	1.5	3.5
Ghana, 2003	95	2.2	2.0	1.8	1.1
Cote d'Ivoire, 2005	97	4.7	3.4	5.3	0.64
Asia and the Caribbean					
India, 2005-06	13‡	0.28	0.22‡	0.37‡	0.59

* All countries for which data are available from national surveys.

† Because many African men are circumcised in their late teens, the table reports circumcision and HIV prevalence by circumcision status for men aged 20 years and above. These percentages are calculated from published data by subtracting data for men aged 15-19 from data for all men.

‡ Including men aged 15-20 years.

Note: For Cote d'Ivoire, India, Malawi, Tanzania, Uganda, and Zimbabwe, data are for men to age 49 years; for Kenya data are for men to age 54 years; for other countries data include men to age 59 years.

Sources: See the Statistical Annex.

Failing to explain high HIV prevalence in women

Because there are a lot of HIV-positive men in generalized epidemics, many women acquire HIV from sexual partners. But sex is not necessarily the whole story. In countries and communities with the worst generalized epidemics, HIV prevalence increases from low levels in women aged 15 years to reach a maximum in women in their late 20s to late 30s (Figure 7.1). In young women, high rates of HIV incidence boost HIV prevalence. However, high rates of incidence are also required to maintain high HIV prevalence in women aged over 25 years.

Consider what happens to women in Lesotho, where a national survey found HIV prevalence over 40 percent for women aged 25 to 39 years. Without treatment, approximately 4 percent of Lesothan women aged 25 to 39 years die of AIDS each year (calculating 10 percent annual mortality among the 40 percent who are HIV-positive). To maintain 40 percent prevalence, another 4 percent of women (or 7 percent of the 60 percent who are HIV-negative) must be newly infected each year. In other words, approximately 7 percent of susceptible (HIV-negative) women aged 25 to 39 years acquire HIV infections each year – a rate that may well be higher than for younger women.

Figure 7.1: HIV prevalence in women by age in Southern Africa

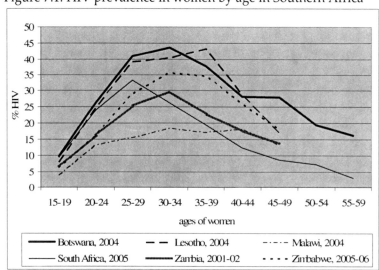

Sources: See the Statistical Annex.

In short, women in the worst generalized epidemics acquire HIV infections at high rates from their late teens at least through their 30s. Moreover, appreciable levels of HIV prevalence – and incidence – continue in older women. A recent study in Gondar, Ethiopia, found 4.7 percent HIV prevalence among women aged 50 to more than 70 years, including two HIV-positive women aged 70 years who had been widowed for 11 years.[47] HIV prevalence in older women in this study exceeded the 1.9 percent prevalence for women aged 15 to 49 years in Ethiopia's 2005 national survey.

Limited sexual risks in young women

Women's sexual risks vary over their lifetime. Before they are married, women are at risk from casual partners, some of whom may become spouses or cohabiting partners. In the worst generalized epidemics, young women who report few sexual partners are nevertheless at high risk for infection. For example, in Carletonville, South Africa, in 1999, sexually active women aged 16-18 years reported an average of 1.7 sexual partners in their life (almost all casual), and few sexual contacts per partnership – yet 21 percent were HIV-positive.[48] Similarly, in Kisumu, Kenya, in 1997-98, 20 percent of unmarried women less than 20 years old who reported only one lifetime sexual partner were HIV-positive.[49]

Various hypotheses have been proposed to explain how the limited sexual activity reported by young women in many African communities could account for their observed high rates of HIV prevalence. One is that women have sex with older men, who are more likely to be HIV-positive than younger men. Another is that younger vs. older women have much greater biological susceptibility to sexual acquisition of HIV. None of these hypotheses has been rigorously tested by tracing casual partners that are alleged to infect young women. Also, the challenge to understand generalized epidemics is to explain high incidence in women at least through their 30s, not only in young women.

Limited sexual risks in older women

Between the ages of 25 and 50 years, most women in Africa and in other countries with generalized epidemics are married, and most married women report no non-spousal partners. Nevertheless, in nine of 17 countries with generalized epidemics and with available data from national surveys, more than half of HIV-positive married women had HIV-negative husbands (Table 7.5). Because HIV transmission can go both ways, some women with HIV-positive husbands no doubt infected their husbands, rather than the other way around. Furthermore, even when both partners are HIV-positive, wives and husbands may have acquired their infections from different outside sources. Studies in Zambia and Malawi that sequenced HIV from couples in which both partners were HIV-positive found dissimilar HIV and therefore unlinked infections in 13 percent and 28 percent of couples, respectively.[50]

Table 7.5: HIV infection in couples in countries with generalized epidemics*

Country	HIV in couples (% of couples)			% of married HIV+ women with HIV- partners
	Both HIV+	Wife only HIV+	Husband only HIV+	
Africa				
Burkina Faso, 2003	0.3	0.7	0.7	70
Cameroon, 2004	2.4	2.7	2.4	53
Cote d'Ivoire, 2005	1.4	3.7	2.3	73
Ethiopia, 2005	0.3	1.0	0.8	77
Ghana, 2003	1.0	1.5	1.6	60
Guinea, 2005	0.4	0.7	1.0	64
Kenya, 2003	3.7	4.6	2.8	55
Lesotho, 2004	20.2	4.5	8.9	18
Malawi, 2004	7.0	4.0	5.7	36
Niger, 2006	0.2	0.4	0.6	67
Rwanda, 2005	1.7	0.8	1.4	32
Tanzania, 2003	2.6	3.5	4.4	57
Uganda, 2004-05	3.4	1.8	2.8	35
Zimbabwe, 2005-06	14.7	5.2	8.1	26
Asia and the Caribbean				
Cambodia, 2005-06	0.5	0.1	0.4	17
Haiti, 2005	1.5	1.2	2.0	44
India, 2005-06	0.11	0.07	0.32	39

* All countries for which data are available from national surveys.
Sources: See the Statistical Annex.

A recent World Bank paper interprets the high proportion of HIV-positive wives with HIV-negative husbands in national surveys in Africa as evidence that 'extramarital sexual activity among cohabiting women...is a substantial source of vulnerability to HIV,' and that 'self-reported sexual behaviors are not very reliable.'[51] Some women no doubt misreport the number of their sexual partners. But to simply assume and assert that HIV-positive women with HIV-negative partners acquired their infections from extramarital liaisons is not only bad science, but also dangerous for women. What the World Bank has done in publishing such unsupported allegations is equivalent to the town gossip and troublemaker telling husbands – without evidence – that their wives are fooling around.

Both the popular and the scholarly AIDS literature are full of anecdotes of philandering HIV-positive spouses, poverty-driven sex work, and sugar-daddies. But these anecdotes do not describe the reality for most HIV-positive women in generalized epidemics. The 'average' HIV-positive woman has had few pre-marital partners and few or no extra-marital partners, has had a sufficiently high social status that she was not driven to trade sex for favors, and has – often – an HIV-negative husband. What's missing?

Extending a metaphor

AIDS researchers in Africa have been like traffic safety experts who persistently analyze accidents with the limiting assumption that all traffic on a two-way street comes exclusively from one direction. After decades, such traffic safety experts are still arguing and hypothesizing about why some intersections are many times more dangerous than others, and are still refusing to take a good look at how much traffic might be coming from the other direction.

Single-minded attention to sex in HIV research contributed to single-minded attention to sex in HIV prevention messages. These messages – supported by billions of dollars in foreign aid – promote the stigmatizing assumption that an adult's HIV infection is a reliable sign of sexual exposure.

---

[1] 'Constitution of the World Health Organization.' *Bull WHO* 2002; 80: 984.

[2] Stillwagon E. *AIDS and the Ecology of Poverty*. Oxford: Oxford University Press, 2006. p. 135.

[3] Rushton JP, Bogaert AF. 'Population differences in susceptibility to AIDS: An evolutionary analysis', *Soc Sci Med*, 1989, 28: 1211-20.

[4] Packard RM, Epstein P. 'Epidemiologists, social scientists, and the structure of medical research on AIDS in Africa', *Soc Sci Med*, 1991, 33: 771-83. p. 781.

[5] Cleland J, Ferry B, Carael M. 'Summary and conclusions', in Cleland J, Ferry B (eds). *Sexual behavior and AIDS in the developing world*. Geneva: WHO, 1995, pp. 208-28. p. 211.

[6] Wellings K, Collumbien M, Slaymaker E, et al. 'Sexual behavior in context: A global perspective', *Lancet*, 2006, 368: 1706-28. p. 1723.

[7] Chin J. *The AIDS Pandemic: The collision of epidemiology with political correctness*. Abingdon, UK: Radcliffe, 2007. pp 146-7.

[8] Panos Institute. *The 3rd Epidemic: Repercussions of the Fear of AIDS*. London: Panos Publications, 1990. p. i.

[9] Garnett GP, Fraser C. 'Let it be sexual – Selection, aggregation and distortion used to construct a case against sexual transmission [letter]', *Int J STD AIDS*, 2003, 14: 782-4. p. 782.

[10] Gray R, Thoma M, Kiwanuka N, et al. 'HIV transmission through health care in sub-Saharan Africa, authors' replies [letter]', *Lancet*, 2004, 364: 1666.

[11] Frerichs RR. 'Personal screening for HIV in developing countries', *Lancet*, 1994, 343: 960-2.

[12] Mertens TE, Smith GD, Van Praag E. 'Home testing for HIV [letter]', *Lancet*, 1994, 343: 1293.

[13] WHO. *The Health Sector Response to HIV/AIDS: Coverage of selected services in 2001*. Geneva: WHO, 2002.

[14] Great Britain, House of Commons (Session 2000-2001), International Development Committee. *Third Report, HIV/AIDS: The impact on social and economic development*, vol. 2 (HC 354-II). London: House of Commons, 2001. Evidence of Peter Piot on 18 July 2000.

[15] Stringer EM, Sinkala M, Kumwenda R, et al. 'Personal risk perception, HIV knowledge and risk avoidance behavior, and their relationships to actual HIV serostatus in an urban African obstetric population', *J Acquir Immune Defic Syndr*, 2004, 35: 60-6.

[16] Correa M, Gisselquist D. *HIV from Blood Exposures in India – An exploratory study*. Colombo: Norwegian Church Aid, 2005. p. 51.

[17] Public Health Service (PHS). 'Policy on informing those tested about HIV serostatus.' Washington, DC: PHS, 1988. Available at: http://www.hhs.gov/ohrp/humansubjects/guidance/hsdc88jun.htm (accessed 9 September 2007).

[18] Allen SA, Karita E, N'gandu N, et al. 'The evolution of voluntary testing and counseling as an HIV prevention strategy', in Gibney L, DiClemente RJ, Vermund SH, (eds). *Preventing HIV in Developing Countries: Biomedical and behavioral approaches*. New York: Kluwer Academic, 1999. pp. 87-108. p. 103.

[19] Gray RH, Wawer MJ, Brookmeyer R, et al. 'Probability of HIV-1 transmission per coital act in monogamous, heterosexual, HIV-1 discordant couples in Rakai, Uganda', *Lancet*, 2001, 357: 1149-53. p. 1152.

[20] Quinn TC, Wawer MJ, Sewankambo N, et al. 'Viral load and heterosexual transmission of human immunodeficiency virus type 1', *N Engl J Med*, 2000, 342: 921-9.

[21] Hugonnet S, Mosha F, Todd J, et al. 'Incidence of HIV infection in stable sexual partnerships: A retrospective cohort study of 1802 couples in Mwanza Region, Tanzania', *J Acquir Immune Defic Syndr*, 2002, 30: 73-80. p. 77.

[22] Humphrey JH, Iliff PJ, Marinda ET, et al. 'Effects of a single large dose of vitamin A, given during the postpartum period to HIV-positive women and their infants, on child HIV infection, HIV-free survival, and mortality', *J Infect Dis*, 2006, 193: 860-71; Marinda E, Humphrey JH, Iliff PJ, et al. 'Child mortality according to maternal and infant HIV status in Zimbabwe', *Ped Infect Dis J*, 2007, 26: 519-26.

[23] Piwocz EG, Iliff PJ, Tavengwa N, et al. 'An education and counseling program for preventing breast-feeding-associated HIV transmission in Zimbabwe: design and impact on maternal knowledge and behavior', *J Nutr*, 2005, 135: 950-5. p. 951.

[24] Humphrey JH et al. 'Effects of a single large dose of vitamin A'.

[25] Gray RH et al. 'Probability of HIV-1 transmission per coital act'; Gray RH, Wabwire-Mangen F, Kigozi G, et al. 'Randomized trial of presumptive sexually transmitted disease therapy during pregnancy in Rakai, Uganda', *Am J Obstet Gynecol*, 2001, 185: 1209-17.

[26] Hugonnet S et al. 'Incidence of HIV infection in stable sexual partnerships'.

[27] Humphrey JH et al. 'Effects of a single large dose of vitamin A'.

[28] 'Nuremberg Code.' Available from: http://www.hhs.gov/ohrp/irb/irb_appendices.htm#j5 (accessed 9 September 2007).

[29] 'World Medical Association Declaration of Helsinki.' Available from: www.wma.net/e/policy/b3.htm (accessed 9 September 2007).

[30] Gavin L, Galavotti C, Dube H, et al. 'Factors associated with HIV infection in adolescent females in Zimbabwe', *J Adolesc Health*, 2006, 39: 596.e11-18.

[31] Rehle T, Shisana O, Pillay V, et al. 'National HIV incidence measures – New insights into the South African epidemic', *S Afr Med J*, 2007, 97: 194-9.

[32] Lopman BA, Garnett GP, Mason PR, et al. 'Individual level injection history: A lack of association with HIV incidence in rural Zimbabwe', *PLoS Med*, 2005, 2(2): e37.

[33] Rehle T et al. 'National HIV incidence measures'.

[34] Allen S, Tice J, Van de Perre P, et al. 'Effect of serotesting with counselling on condom use and seroconversion among HIV discordant couples in Africa', *BMJ*, 1992, 304: 1605-9; Lopman BA et al. 'Individual level injection history'.

[35] Auvert B, Taljaard D, Lagarde E, et al. 'Randomized, controlled intervention trial of male circumcision for reduction of HIV infection risk: The ANRS 1265 trial', *PLoS Med*, 2005, 2: e298.

[36] Gray RH, Kigozi G, Serwadda D, et al. 'Male circumcision for HIV prevention in men in Rakai, Uganda: a randomized trial', *Lancet*, 2007, 369: 657-66.

[37] Bailey RC, Moses S, Parkere CB, et al. 'Male circumcision for HIV prevention in young men in Kisumu, Kenya: a randomised controlled trial', *Lancet*, 2007, 369: 643-56.

[38] Brewer D, Potterat JJ, Roberts JM, Brody S. 'Male and female circumcision associated with prevalent HIV infection in virgins and adolescents in Kenya, Lesotho, and Tanzania', *Ann Epidemiol*, 2007, 17: 217-26.

[39] Gray RH, Li X, Kigozi G, et al. 'Increased risk of incident HIV during pregnancy in Rakai, Uganda: a prospective study', *Lancet*, 2005, 366: 1182-8.

[40] Gray RH et al. 'Randomized trial of presumptive sexually transmitted disease therapy'.

[41] CDC. 'Antiretroviral postexposure prophylaxis after sexual, injection drug-use, or other nonoccupational exposure to HIV in the United States: Recommendations from the US Department of Health and Human Services', *MMWR*, 2005, 54 (No. RR-2): 1-20; Gray RH et al. 'Probability of HIV-1 transmission per coital act'.

[42] Gisselquist D, Potterat JJ. 'Heterosexual transmission of HIV in Africa: An empiric estimate', *Int J STD AIDS*, 2003, 14: 162-73.

[43] Wawer MJ, Sewankambo NK, Serwadda D, et al. 'Control of sexually transmitted diseases for AIDS prevention in Uganda: A randomized community trial', *Lancet*, 1999, 353: 525-535; Kamali A, Quigley M, Nakiyingi J, et al. 'Syndromic management of sexually-transmitted infections and behaviour change interventions on transmission of HIV-1 in rural Uganda: a community randomized trial', *Lancet*, 2003, 361: 645-52; Gisselquist D, Potterat JJ, Brody S. 'Running on empty: Sexual co-factors are insufficient to fuel Africa's turbo-charged HIV epidemic', *Int J STD AIDS*, 2004, 15: 442-52.

[44] Epstein H. *The Invisible Cure*. New York: Farrar, Straus and Giroux, 2007; Chin J. *The AIDS Pandemic*.

[45] Lagarde L, Auvert B, Carael M, et al. 'Concurrent sexual partnerships and HIV prevalence in five urban communities of sub-Saharan Africa', *AIDS*, 2001, 15: 877-84.

[46] Bongaarts J, Reining P, Way P, et al. 'The relationship between male circumcision and HIV infection in African populations', *AIDS*, 1989, 3: 373-7; Moses S, Bradley JE, Nagelkerke NJD, et al. 'Geographical patterns of male circumcision practices in Africa: Association with HIV seroprevalence', *Int J Epidemiol*, 1990, 19: 693-7.

[47] Kassu A, Mekonnen A, Bekele A, et al. 'HIV and syphilis infection among elderly people in northwest Ethiopia', *Jpn J Infect Dis*, 2004, 57: 264-7.

[48] Auvert B, Ballard R, Campbell C, et al. 'HIV infection among youth in a South African mining town is associated with herpes simplex virus-2 seropositivity and sexual behaviour', *AIDS*, 2001, 15: 885-98.

147

[49] Glynn JR, Carael M, Auvert B, et al. 'Why do young women have a much higher prevalence of HIV than young men? A study in Kisumu, Kenya and Ndola, Zambia, *AIDS*, 2001, 15 (suppl 4): S51-60.

[50] Fideli US, Allen SA, Musonda R, et al. 'Virologic and immunologic determinants of heterosexual transmission of human immunodeficiency virus type 1 in Africa', *AIDS Res Hum Retroviruses*, 2001, 17: 901-10; McCormack GP, Glynn JR, Crampin AC, et al. 'Early evolution of the human immunodeficiency virus type 1 subtype C epidemic in rural Malawi', *J Virol*, 2002, 76: 12890-9.

[51] de Walque D. 'Discordant couples: HIV infection among couples in Burkina Faso, Cameroon, Ghana, Kenya, and Tanzania', World Bank Policy Research Working Paper 3956. Washington DC: World Bank, 2006. pp. 1, 18.

Chapter 8

HOW MUCH HIV INFECTION COMES FROM BLOOD EXPOSURES?

What proportion of HIV infections in countries with generalized epidemics comes from blood exposures (except IDU and blood transfusions)? When infection control in health care is not routine and reliable, the answer to this question is both important and not immediately obvious.

Two preliminary issues

HIV survival outside the body

Laboratory studies through 1988 showed that HIV survives outside the body at room temperature for a few hours to a few days when dry, and for several weeks when wet (see Chapter 5). Several studies after 1988 show that 10 percent of an initial deposit of HIV can survive in dry conditions – such as on a glass slide – for several hours to more than a day.[1] Research published in 1999 showed that HIV can survive for weeks at room temperature in wet conditions, such as in a used syringe or needle.[2] Wiping or rinsing does not reliably remove or kill (inactivate) HIV. Except in carefully controlled conditions, even soaking contaminated instruments in bleach or alcohol does not reliably kill HIV, because fluids might not penetrate clots or small spaces in syringes and needles, solutions might weaken over time, and presence of organic matter interferes with bleach.[3] Heating to boiling reliably kills HIV. Soaking in glutaraldehyde or other special chemicals is also effective.

Many public health experts understate HIV survival. For example, the *British Medical Journal* in 2007 quoted a 'senior research scientist' at Harvard's School of Public Health to say, 'The HIV virus is extremely fragile, dying easily and quickly once exposed to air.'[4] Similarly, web-based training materials for nurses posted by Johns Hopkins aver that 'HIV cannot live outside body fluids more than a few seconds.' and that 'HIV can live between 30 seconds to one minute when exposed to the air.'[5] These statements are not only dead wrong, they are deadly.

149

Risk to transmit HIV through trace amounts of blood

In a 1991 article, senior officials in WHO's Global Programme on AIDS estimated that the risk to transmit HIV from an HIV-positive patient to a subsequent patient through reused 'equipment/needles' was less than 0.5 percent.[6] Because this is an important estimate, it is useful to look at relevant evidence.

A 1991 review of risks to transmit HIV through health care averred that needlestick injuries to healthcare workers 'give an idea of the risk of transmission from non-intravenous injection of blood and suggest that this is not an efficient mode of transmission.'[7] Through 1996, evidence compiled from multiple studies that followed healthcare workers exposed to HIV through needlestick accidents showed that only 20 (0.3 percent) of 6,202 acquired HIV infections.[8]

However, the parallel does not fit. In the mid-1990s, CDC looked at what was different about needlestick accidents that led to HIV infections vs. those that did not. Not surprisingly, deep needlesticks – deep enough for the hole of the needle to be within the skin, as in an injection – were much more dangerous than shallow scratches. And only 7 percent of needlestick accidents were deep. With data from this study, the average risk for a healthcare worker to acquire HIV infection from a deep needlestick can be estimated at 2.3 percent.[9]

Thus, based on information from needlestick accidents, a good first estimate of the risk to transmit HIV from patient to patient through syringes and needles reused without sterilization is 2.3 percent. However, many other factors – presence of visible blood, whether the needle came from a vein, the size of the needle – raise or lower this risk. If HIV contaminates multidose vials or rinsing pans, HIV may spread from one patient to infect more than one subsequent patient. Rinsing or washing syringes or needles without sterilization may lower the risk.

Other estimates of the risk to transmit HIV through trace amounts of blood come from studies among IDUs. Two studies in New Haven, US, and in Bangkok, Thailand, used information from IDUs to estimate the risk to transmit HIV through a single intravenous injection with shared and contaminated equipment. These estimates are 0.67 percent and 0.8 percent in the US and Thailand, respectively.[10] However, both studies rejected IDUs' statements about how often they shared injection equipment, and assumed instead that many if not most shared more often than they reported. The researchers also assumed that all sharing was random, with an 'average' IDU. If the researchers had used reported rather than assumed rates of sharing, and had considered that IDUs who share often do so with regular partners, their estimated risks to transmit HIV through injections would have been much higher.

The best evidence on risks to pass HIV from patient to patient through invasive healthcare procedures comes from hospital-based outbreaks where that has happened on a large scale. What one needs to know to calculate the risk is the average numbers of invasive procedures (and details about the procedures) administered to HIV-positive persons that result in one HIV transmission to another patient. Unfortunately, no one has reported sufficiently detailed information from any large nosocomial outbreak to calculate the risk. However, there is enough information to make some rough estimates.

For example, in southern Russia in 1988-89, invasive procedures at 13 hospitals passed HIV from one child directly and indirectly (through other children) to more than 260 children over 15 months (Chapter 9 provides more information on this outbreak).[11] Most transmissions during this outbreak came from inpatient children who themselves had been infected not more than six weeks earlier.[12] If we assume that the risk to transmit HIV through healthcare was constant throughout the outbreak, and that each infected child infected an average of 1-2 children over 1-2 months, this would produce the observed nosocomial infections.

With this model, how many procedures did HIV-positive children have over one month to infect one other child? No one has reported this information, but a rough estimate is possible. If HIV-positive children had an average of 10-50 procedures per month, after which instruments were subsequently reused without sterilization, the calculated average risk to transmit HIV per procedure would be 2 percent to 10 percent. Similar rough estimates can be derived from several other documented nosocomial outbreaks.[13]

What proportion of HIV infections comes from blood exposures?

Some people propose that blood exposures (except transfusions and IDU) account for as little as 0.01 percent of HIV infections in the world, while others have estimated that blood exposures account for more than 50 percent of infections in generalized epidemics. One way to approach the debate is to distinguish between weaker and stronger evidence, and to consider what additional evidence could be collected to settle the matter.

Estimates based on no evidence and/or indirect evidence

As discussed in Chapter 5, experts consulted by WHO in 1988 estimated that 'inadequately sterilized skin-piercing instruments (health sector and outside)' accounted for 1.6 percent of HIV infections in Africa.[14] The paper that reports this estimate provides no calculations or argument linking it to any evidence. In 1991, senior officials in WHO's Global Programme on AIDS proposed that 'equipment/needles' accounted for less than 0.1 percent of HIV infections in Africa, again without presenting any supporting evidence.[15]

A 1991 review acknowledged that 'the proportion of HIV infection transmitted parenterally [though skin-piercing procedures] has not been well studied,' but estimated nonetheless that medical injections accounted for not more than 'occasional transmission of HIV' in Africa. To reach this conclusion, the review relied heavily on indirect evidence, arguing that 'injections in the 5-14-year age group are very common, yet cases of HIV infection and AIDS in this age group are relatively rare.'[16] This common argument not only discounts studies that report appreciable numbers of unexplained HIV infections in children, but also relies on the invalid assumption that adults' risks for nosocomial HIV infection would be not much greater than children's risks (see Chapter 5).

Estimates from models using numbers of unsafe injections

In 1999 and 2004, two WHO teams published estimates of the number of HIV infections from medical injections, calculated from survey-based estimates of the number of unsafe injections. According to these estimates, 2-5 percent of new HIV infections in the world were from unsafe injections.

To see how these estimates are derived, consider the calculations that produced the first such estimate in 1999.[17] (This explanation follows the logic of the model, but simplifies the calculations.) Briefly, the WHO team estimated that 20 million Africans were HIV-positive. They also estimated (from surveys in several African countries) that Africans received 1-2 injections per year, and they assumed that HIV-positive Africans received the same number of injections as did other Africans. Hence, each year, doctors and others administered 20-40 million injections to HIV-positive patients. Next, from surveys of injection practices, the models estimated that doctors reused syringes without sterilization after 50 percent of all injections, and thereby after 10-20 million injections administered to HIV-positive patients.

But here comes the crucial assumption: the WHO team assumed that only 0.5 percent of patients who received injections with HIV-contaminated syringes or needles (that is, with equipment reused without sterilization after injecting an HIV-positive patient) contracted HIV infections. Thus, the model calculated that 0.5 percent of 10-20 million Africans – approximately 50,000-100,000 people – contracted HIV each year from injections. If the WHO team had used a higher rate of HIV transmission through reused equipment – such as the 2.3 percent average risk of transmission to healthcare workers through deep needlestick accidents – their calculations would have 'found' many more HIV infections.

As of 2006, UNAIDS[18] accepted the estimate from WHO's later model-based calculation that medical injections account for 5 percent of HIV infections in the world.[19] These estimates focus on injections. Other blood exposures taken together – drawing blood, tattooing, minor surgeries, etc – might be more common and more damaging than injections. But even with good information about the numbers of unsafe procedures, model-based estimates are unreliable. Their weakness is that they depend on an assumed – not an observed – rate of HIV transmission per event.

Estimates from studies of risks for incident HIV infection

Compared to models, studies of risks for incident HIV infection – studies that follow HIV-negative people, retest them to see who becomes HIV-positive, and ask about sex and blood exposures – are able to provide more reliable estimates of the proportion of HIV infections coming from health care.

In 2001, UNAIDS commissioned Nicole Seguy to review studies of risks for HIV infection that asked about medical injections. She found four studies in Africa that followed and tested people in the general population, and asked about injections as risks for incident infections. Her 5 September 2002 draft concluded that these studies showed that 'contaminated injections may cause between 12 percent and 33 percent of new HIV infections' in Africa.[20] UNAIDS did not publish the paper.

Table 8.1: Estimates of the proportion of incident HIV infections from injections

Country, year of study	Population	Relative risk for HIV in persons reporting any vs no injections	% of HIV infections 'attributable' to injections*
Studies included in Seguy's review			
DRC, Kinshasa, 1984-86[21]	Healthcare workers	1.5	28
Uganda, Rakai, 1989-90[22]	Adults	1.1	8.5
Rwanda, Butare, 1989-93[23]	Women	2.4	45
Uganda, Masaka, 1990-97[24]	Men	5.2	41
	Women	1.6	16
Other results			
Rwanda, Butare, 1989-93[25]	Women	1.2	11
Uganda, Masaka, 1990-2005[26]	Adults	8.5	29
Tanzania, Mwanza, 1991-94[27]	Men	1.7	23
	Women	1.4	19
Uganda, Rakai, 1997-99[28]	Adults	1.0	1.5†
Zimbabwe, Manicaland, 1999-03[29]	Men	<1	<0
	Women	1.3	12

* This column reports the crude population attributable fractions (PAFs) of incident infections associated with injections. These PAFs are calculated from the ratio of the rates (RR) of HIV incidence in persons who reported vs. persons who did not report injections, and the proportion (ϱ) of people with incident infections who reported injections, using the formula: PAF = $\varrho(RR-1)/RR$. For more information about PAFs see standard epidemiology texts.
† This result appears to be based on a subset of adults selected from a larger study.[30]

During 2004-07, other studies reported additional information on injections as risks for incident HIV infection in Africa. Taking all of these studies together, 11 of 12 results show that men and/or women who reported injections were more likely to show up with a new HIV infection as compared to those who reported no injections (Table 8.1). Reporting an injection increased their risk to acquire an HIV infection by as much as 8.5 times, with a median increase of 1.5 times. Using standard analyses to link HIV infections to injections (see notes to Table 8.1), these studies attribute as much as 45 percent (median 21 percent) of new HIV infections to injections. (These analyses measure the 'extra' infections in people who report injections vs. people who do not, but do not prove that injections caused these infections.)

A handful of studies have examined other blood exposures as risks for incident HIV infections. For example, in Pune, India, during 1993-2000 new infections were more common in people who had received a tattoo.[31] In addition, some studies of risks for prevalent HIV infection which have taken care to exclude reverse causation (that is, to exclude healthcare procedures solicited by people to treat HIV-related symptoms) provide relevant evidence. For example, a study of healthy Zambian women (with no symptoms suggesting HIV infection) found that women reporting any vs. no injections in the past 5 years were 2.6 times more likely to be HIV-positive;[32] and a study in Zanzibar, Tanzania, found that HIV prevalence was 1.9 times greater in those who reported having had an operation vs. those who reported no operations.[33]

Studies not done

The best way to determine the proportion of HIV infections from various risks is to trace infections to their source. In countries with generalized epidemics, some studies have traced a minority of infections to spouses. But only rarely has an infection been traced to any other source, leaving too much room for speculation.

Initial vs. total impact on HIV epidemic expansion

All the above estimates measure only the direct contribution of blood exposures to HIV epidemics, which is less than the total – direct plus indirect – contribution. Suppose, for example, that 10 percent of people with new HIV infections in Zambia during 1989-2007 acquired their infections directly from injections. Many of these 10 percent would subsequently transmit HIV to others through sex and/or blood, and these others would in turn transmit through multiple modes, and so on. Thus, the direct plus indirect contribution of HIV transmission through injections during 1989-2007 on the number of infections in Zambia in 2007 would be far greater than 10 percent.

Moreover, HIV transmission through blood exposures accelerates sexual transmission by allowing HIV to jump from one sexual network to others. If, for example, a husband and wife are both HIV-positive and have no other sex partners, their HIV has no chance to reach anyone through sex. But if the husband transmits HIV to someone through a dental clinic, the HIV can get into another sexual network, where sexual transmission again becomes possible.

WHO, UNAIDS, and allies repeat low estimates

Seguy's unpublished paper along with several articles published in 2002-03[34] challenged WHO's and UNAIDS's lack of attention to HIV transmission through health care. In response, WHO and UNAIDS staff led a group of 15 authors in a review defending WHO's low estimates of HIV infections from healthcare.[35]

Their review, published in 2004, did not mention Seguy's unpublished draft. Moreover, at least some of the authors were aware of – and did not report – unpublished data from Masaka, Uganda, and from Mwanza, Tanzania, which linked more than 20 percent of incident HIV infections to injections. The Mwanza team did not report these data until 2006, and the Masaka team did not do so until 2007 (see Table 8.1). While not reporting conflicting evidence from studies of risks for incident HIV infection, the authors relied on indirect evidence – including low HIV prevalence in children in selected studies – to defend WHO's low estimates of HIV infections from injections.

Many organizations involved in HIV prevention in generalized epidemics have continued to use unsupported low estimates for the proportion of HIV infection from blood exposures. For example, USAID, in a 2002 document, attributed only 0.01 percent of global HIV infections to health care (except blood transfusions).[36] And WHO's 2002 World Health Report ignored WHO's own model-based estimates to say, 'Current estimates suggest that more than 99% of the HIV infections prevalent in Africa in 2001 are attributable to unsafe sex.'[37]

Not only HIV: Other bloodborne viruses

Hepatitis B virus

In much of Africa and Asia, 70-95 percent of adults have been infected with hepatitis B virus at some time in their lives, and 8-20 percent have active (chronic or new) infections. Childhood acquisition of hepatitis B, which often leads to lifetime chronic infection, accounts for most active hepatitis B infections in Africa.

For several decades after tests for hepatitis B were available, no researcher looking at risks for hepatitis B infection in African children reported information on injections.[38] The first study to do so tested children aged 6 months to 5 years from seven villages in Gambia in 1988, and then followed and retested them in 1990. The baseline survey in 1988 reported no association between hepatitis B infection and 'number of injections for immunization.'[39] The study, unfortunately, did not report the relevant data (which might have shown more immunizations for infected children, but with more than a 5 percent chance that the observation was a statistical accident). The study also did not report any information about curative injections.

The follow-up study found that 30 percent of susceptible children (setting aside children who had past or current infections in the baseline survey) had contracted hepatitis B infections over two years. The study reported a 'slight excess of injections recorded by infected children: 0.82...versus 0.66...in uninfected children.'[40] Assuming that each child had received 0 or 1 injection, and using standard analyses, these reported data are consistent with injections accounting for more than a third of new infections. The study also reported large unexplained differences in hepatitis B incidence between villages – with incidence over two years ranging from 21 percent to 54 percent. The study did not consider that such differences might have been due to differences in infection control practices on the part of the clinics and healthcare workers serving the different villages, and the study reported nothing about infection control practices.

With few exceptions, researchers in Africa continued to avoid, ignore, or deny evidence that healthcare is a risk for hepatitis B infection. They continued, at the same time, to come up with no explanation for high rates of infection in African children or adults. For example, the Gambian study mentioned in the previous paragraph found that 'insecticide spraying of the child's dwelling...[reduced] exposure to bedbugs but there was no effect on hepatitis B infection.'[41] A 1993 review of hepatitis B in Africa acknowledged, 'The phenomenon of horizontal [child-to-child] transmission of HBV [hepatitis B virus] has never been adequately explained.'[42]

In contrast, researchers in Asia and Eastern Europe looked at healthcare risks for hepatitis B and were more successful in both explaining and curbing high rates of infection. For example, when researchers in China found that 21 percent of children aged 1 year had active hepatitis B infections, they noted that healthcare workers changed needles but reused syringes without sterilization. Healthcare managers responded with 'stricter measures...to prevent HBV [hepatitis B virus] infection in these clinics, including training of medical personnel...and the use of sterilized syringes and needles for single injections.'[43] With these changes, the prevalence of active hepatitis B infection among children aged 1 year whose mothers were not infected (to exclude mother-to-child transmission) fell from 15 to 3.3 percent.

During 1999 to 2004, the same WHO teams that modeled the contribution of medical injections to HIV infections (using survey-based estimates of the number of unsafe injections) also modeled the contribution of injections to hepatitis B infections. According to the latest estimate from 2004, injections account for only 10 percent of hepatitis B infections in Africa.[44] Considering that IDUs and MSMs contribute little to hepatitis B transmission in Africa – and certainly not among children – this estimate is very likely low.

Hepatitis B vaccine was introduced in 1981. Most countries have begun to vaccinate infants against hepatitis B. Preventing hepatitis B infection in infants and young children prevents most new chronic infections.

Hepatitis C virus

WHO estimates much higher prevalence of hepatitis C virus infection in Africa than in developed countries.[45] Although hepatitis C transmits almost exclusively through blood exposures, few studies in Africa have identified the blood exposures that transmit hepatitis C. A large majority of studies in Africa that have tested people for both hepatitis C and HIV find that HIV infection is more common in people with hepatitis C virus or antibodies.[46] Because IDUs have been rare in

Africa, this points to other blood exposures transmitting both HIV and hepatitis C.

Low prevalence of hepatitis C virus or antibodies in Southern Africa – lower even than in Western Europe or the US – presents a puzzle. This low prevalence has been presented as evidence that blood exposures are not common in Southern Africa, and therefore that HIV acquisition among adults in the region must be almost entirely through sex.[47] However, much remains unknown about hepatitis C in Africa, and more generally about people's ability to resist and to defeat hepatitis C infection.

Recent studies suggest that many people who have been infected with the hepatitis C virus defeat it within several months, and do not subsequently carry antibodies. For example, 8 of 116 US health care workers exposed to hepatitis C through needlestick accidents became at least transiently infected – determined by finding the virus in their blood – but only 2 of 8 developed antibodies, and only 1 of 8 (1 of the 2 with antibodies) developed a chronic infection.[48] Also, some people defeat chronic infections over time, and some who do subsequently lose antibodies.

The ability to resist or to defeat hepatitis C infections may vary by age, virus type, and other factors. Notably, the hepatitis C virus type that circulates in Southern Africa – type 5 – is rare outside the region.[49] Thus, low prevalence of hepatitis C infection and antibodies in Southern Africa does not reliably show the proportion of people who have been exposed to hepatitis C or to other bloodborne viruses – and does not, therefore, show that sex accounts for most HIV infections in Southern Africa.

Ebola, Marburg, and Lassa virus outbreaks

Ebola, Marburg, and Lassa viruses – all of which cause viral hemorrhagic fever – circulate over large areas of Africa among non-human hosts. All three occasionally infect humans. Some infections may be unnoticed or mild, while others lead to pain, fever, bleeding, and often death. Person-to-person transmission outside hospitals appears to be too inefficient – too infrequent – to sustain an epidemic.

In the last several decades, hospitals in Africa have from time to time spread rare infections of these bloodborne viruses in short but deadly outbreaks. The viruses appear to be most deadly when spread through blood, such as through syringes and needles reused for injections.[50] After the first three documented Ebola outbreaks during 1976-79 (see Chapter 3), no one recognized any new infections in Africa for more than a decade. Ebola returned in 1994-96, causing several outbreaks in Gabon with a total of almost 100 deaths, and a large outbreak with more than 250 deaths in Kikwit, DRC.[51] Another large outbreak in Uganda in 2000-01 caused several hundred deaths.[52] During 2001-03, five Ebola outbreaks in Gabon and Congo led to a combined total of more than 260 deaths,[53] and another outbreak emerged in south-central DRC in 2007.

Two hospitals in Nigeria transmitted Lassa virus during an outbreak in 1995. According to an international team, 'Compelling, indirect evidence revealed that parenteral [skin-piercing] drug rounds with sharing of syringes, conducted by minimally educated and supervised staff, fuelled the epidemic among patients.'[54]

The Marburg virus caused an outbreak of hemorrhagic fever in DRC in 1998-2000, and another large outbreak in Angola with more than 300 deaths in 2004-05. More than 75 percent of the early cases in Angola were among children, mostly infants. Infections in children were 'most probably related to needle use, perhaps for vaccines, perhaps from multidose vials.'[55]

A 2005 review of recurrent epidemics of Ebola, Lassa, and Marburg hemorrhagic fever in Africa concluded that[56]

> transmission of blood-borne viruses in medical facilities of all kinds is probably common [across much of Africa]...Indeed, hepatitis C virus (HCV) and human immunodeficiency virus (HIV) may be the viruses most commonly spread by this method. The difference with the haemorrhagic fever viruses is that the consequences...are immediately noticeable, whereas with HCV and HIV it takes years, even decades, for the transmission to be appreciated.

Why don't we know?

During hospital-based outbreaks of Ebola, Lassa, and Marburg infections, people in the community do not need an investigation to see a connection between the hospital and the illness. But because most HIV infections cause no or only minor symptoms for years, people cannot so easily see the link between HIV infection and medical procedures. In the absence of investigations, an antenatal clinic could, for example, infect hundreds of women with HIV over many years without coming under suspicion.

Finding out how HIV infects so many women is crucial to understanding and stopping generalized epidemics. Most studies that have asked women about medical injections as risks for incident HIV infection have found that women reporting injections were more likely to acquire HIV infection (Table 8.1). What is more remarkable, however, is not the evidence that links HIV infection in women to healthcare, but the rarity of such research.

For example, more than 40 percent of women in Botswana aged 25 to 39 years are HIV-positive. Harvard University, CDC, and other foreign organizations fund and advise HIV research in Botswana. Through late 2007, no one has reported research that has asked any Botswanan woman (or man for that matter) about injections or other blood exposures as risks for HIV infection. Sexual acquisition of HIV infection is assumed.

---

[1] van Bueren J, Simpson RA, Jacobs P, et al. 'Survival of human immunodeficiency virus in suspension and dried onto surfaces', *J Clin Microbiol*, 1994, 32: 571-4; Tjotta E, Humgnes O, Grinde B. 'Survival of HIV-1 activity after disinfection, temperature and pH changes, or drying', *J Med Virol* 1991; 35: 223-7; Kramer A, Schwebke I, Kampf G. 'How long do nosocomial pathogens persist on inanimate surfaces? A systematic review', *BMC Infect Dis*, 2006, 6: 130.

[2] Abdala N, Stephens PC, Griffith BP, et al. 'Survival of HIV-1 in syringes', *J Acquir Immune Defic Syndr*, 1999, 20: 73-80.

[3] Sattar SA, Springthorpe VS. 'Survival and disinfectant inactivation of the human immunodeficiency virus: A critical review. *Rev Infect Dis*, 1991, 13: 430-47; van Bueren J, Simpson RA, Salman H, et al. 'Inactivation of HIV-1 by chemical disinfection: Sodium hypochlorite', *Epidemiol Infect*, 1995, 115: 567-79.

[4] Mosczynski P. 'Unhygienic circumcisions may increase risk of HIV in Africa', *BMJ*, 2007, 334: 498.

[5] Johns Hopkins Center for Clinical Global Health Education (CCGHE). 'Nursing Training Curriculum, HIV Practice and Reducing Stigma, Module I: HIV transmission.' Baltimore: CCGHE, no date. Available at:
http://www.ccghe.jhmi.edu/CCG/distance/HIV_Courses/nurse_training.asp (accessed 9 September 2007). pp. 6, 24.

[6] Heymann DL, Edstrom K. 'Strategies for HIV prevention and control in sub-Saharan Africa', *AIDS*, 1991, 5 (suppl 1): S197-208. p. S197.

[7] Berkley S. 'Parenteral transmission of HIV in Africa', *AIDS*, 1991, 5 (supp 1): S87-92. p. S90.

[8] Bell DM. 'Occupational risk of human immunodeficiency virus infection in healthcare workers: An overview', *Am J Med*, 1997, 102 (suppl 5B): 9-15.

[9] Cardo DM, Culver DH, Ciesielski CA, et al. 'A case-control study of HIV seroconversion in health care workers after percutaneous exposure', *N Eng J Med*, 1997, 337: 1485-90; Gisselquist D, Upham G, Potterat JJ. 'Efficiency of human immunodeficiency virus transmission through injections and other medical procedures: Evidence, estimates, and unfinished business', *Infect Control Hosp Epidemiol*, 2006, 27: 944-52.

[10] Kaplan EH, Heimer R. 'A model-based estimate of HIV infectivity via needle sharing', *J Acquir Immune Defic Syndr*, 1992, 5: 1116-18; Hudgens MG, Longini IM Jr, Halloran ME, et al. 'Estimating the transmission probability of human immunodeficiency virus in injecting drug users in Thailand', *Appl Statist*, 2001, 50: 1-14.

[11] Bobkov A, Garaev MM, Rzhaninova A et al. 'Molecular epidemiology of HIV-1 in the former Soviet Union: Analysis of *env* V3 sequences and their correlation with epidemiologic data', *AIDS*, 1994, 8: 619-24.

[12] Bobkov A, Cheingsong-Popov R, Garaev M, et al. 'Identification of an *env* G subtype and heterogeneity of HIV-1 strains in the Russian Federation and Belarus', *AIDS*, 1994, 8: 1649-55.

[13] Gisselquist D et al. 'Efficiency of human immunodeficiency virus transmission'.

[14] Chin J, Sato PA, Mann JM. 'Projections of HIV infections and AIDS cases to the year 2000', *Bull WHO*, 1990, 68: 1-11. p. 3.

[15] Heymann DL, Edstrom K. 'Strategies for HIV prevention'.

[16] Berkley S. 'Parenteral transmission in Africa'. pp. S87, S90.

[17] Kane A, Lloyd M, Zaffran M, et al. 'Transmission of hepatitis B, hepatitis C and human immunodeficiency viruses through unsafe injections in the developing world: Model-based regional estimates', *Bull WHO*, 1999, 77: 801-7.

[18] UNAIDS. *2006 Report on the Global AIDS Epidemic*. Geneva: UNAIDS, 2006.

[19] Hauri AM, Armstrong GL, Hutin YJF. 'The global burden of disease attributable to contaminated injections given in health care settings', *Int J STD AIDS*. 2004, 15: 7-16.

[20] Randerson J. 'WHO accused of huge HIV blunder', *New Scientist*, 6 December 2003, 180 (2424): 8-9.

[21] N'Galy B, Ryder RW, Bila K, et al. 'Human immunodeficiency virus infection among employees in an African hospital', *N Eng J Med*, 1988, 319: 1123-7.

[22] Wawer MJ, Sewankambo NK, Berkley S, et al. 'Incidence of HIV-1 infection in a rural region of Uganda', *BMJ*, 1994, 308: 171-3.

[23] Bulterys M, Chao A, Habimana P, et al. 'Incident HIV-1 infection in a cohort of young women in Butare, Rwanda', *AIDS*, 1994, 8: 1585-91.

[24] Quigley MA, Morgan D, Malamba SS, et al. 'Case-control study of risk factors for incident HIV infection in rural Uganda', *J Acquir Immune Defic Syndrome*, 2000, 23: 418-25.

[25] Bulterys M, Chao A, Dushimimana A, et al. 'HIV transmission through health care in sub-Saharan Africa, authors' replies [letter]', *Lancet*, 2004, 364: 1665-6.

[26] Whitworth JA, Birao S, Shafer LA, et al. 'HIV incidence and recent injections among adults in rural southwestern Uganda', *AIDS*, 2007, 21: 1056-8.

[27] Todd J, Grosskurth H, Changalucha J, et al. 'Risk factors influencing HIV infection incidence in a rural African population: A nested case-control study', *J Infect Dis*, 2006, 193: 458-66; Gisselquist D. 'New information on the risks of HIV transmission in Mwanza, Tanzania [letter]', *J Infect Dis*, 2006, 194: 536-7.

[28] Kiwanuka N, Gray RH, Serwadda D, et al. 'The incidence of HIV-1 associated with injections and transfusions in a prospective cohort, Rakai, Uganda', *AIDS*, 2004, 18: 342-4.

[29] Lopman BA, Garnett GP, Mason PR, et al. 'Individual level injection history: A lack of association with HIV incidence in rural Zimbabwe', *PLoS Med*, 2005, 2: 142-6.

[30] Gisselquist D. 'HIV transmission through health care in sub-Saharan Africa [letter]', *Lancet*, 2004, 364: 1665.

[31] Reynolds SJ, Risbud AR, Shepherd ME, et al. 'Recent herpes simplex virus type 2 infection and the risk of human immunodeficiency virus type 1 acquisition in India', *J Infect Dis*, 2003, 187: 1513-21.

[32] St Lawrence JS, Klaskala W, Kankasa C, et al. 'Factors associated with HIV prevalence in a pre-partum cohort of Zambian women', *Int J STD AIDS*, 2006, 17: 607-13.

[33] Croce F, Fedeli P, Dahoma M, et al. 'Risk factors for HIV/AIDS in a low HIV prevalence site of sub-Saharan Africa', *Trop Med Int Health*, 2007, 12: 1011-17.

[34] Gisselquist D, Potterat JJ, Brody S, et al. 'Let it be sexual: How health care transmission of AIDS in Africa was ignored', *Int J STD AIDS*, 2003, 14: 148-161; Gisselquist D, Rothenberg R, Potterat JJ, Drucker E. 'HIV infections in sub-Sahara Africa not explained by sexual or vertical transmission', *Int J STD AIDS*, 2002, 13: 657-66.

[35] Schmid GP, Buve A, Mugyenyi P, et al. 'Transmission of HIV-1 infection in sub-Saharan Africa and effect of elimination of unsafe injections', *Lancet*, 2004, 363: 482-8.

[36] USAID. *USAID's Expanded Response to HIV/AIDS*. Washington, DC: USAID, 2002.

[37] WHO. *The World Health Report 2002*. Geneva: WHO, 2002. p. 9.

[38] Hudson C. 'How AIDS forces reappraisal of hepatitis B virus control in sub-Saharan Africa', *Lancet*, 1990, 336: 1364-7.

[39] Mayans MV, Hall AJ, Inskip HM, et al. 'Risk factors for transmission of hepatitis B virus to Gambian children', *Lancet,* 1990, 336: 1107-9. p. 1108.

[40] Mayans MV, Hall AJ, Inskip HM, et al. 'Do bedbugs transmit hepatitis B?', *Lancet,* 1994, 343: 761-3. p. 762.

[41] Ibid. p. 761.

[42] Kiire CF. 'The epidemiology and control of hepatitis B in sub-Saharan Africa', *Prog Med Virol,* 1993, 40: 141-56. p. 146.

[43] Yao GB. 'Importance of perinatal versus horizontal transmission of hepatitis B virus infection in China', *Gut,* 1996; 38 (suppl 2): S39-42. p. S40.

[44] Hauri AM et al. 'The global burden of disease'.

[45] 'Hepatitis C – global prevalence (update)', *Wkly Epidemiol Rec,* 1999, 74: 425-7.

[46] Gisselquist D, Perrin L, Minkin SF. 'Parallel and overlapping HIV and bloodborne hepatitis epidemics in Africa', *Int J STD AIDS,* 2004, 15: 145-52.

[47] Walker PR, Worobey M, Rambaut A, et al. 'Sexual transmission of HIV in Africa', *Nature,* 2003, 422: 679.

[48] Personal communication from Jonathan Schwartz, 23 August 2007.

[49] Davis GL. 'Hepatitis C virus genotypes and quasispecies', *Am J Med,* 1999, 106 (suppl 6B): 21S-26S.

[50] Peters CJ. 'Marburg and Ebola – Arming ourselves against the deadly filoviruses', *N Eng J Med,* 2005, 352: 2571-3.

[51] Colebunders R, Borchert M. 'Ebola haemorrhagic fever – A review', *J Infect,* 2000, 40: 16-20; Khan AS, Tshioko FK, Heymann DL, et al. 'The reemergence of Ebola hemorrhagic fever, Democratic Republic of the Congo, 1995', *J Infect Dis,* 1999, 179 (suppl 1): S76-86.

[52] Okware SI, Omaswa FG, Zaramba S, et al. 'An outbreak of Ebola in Uganda', *Trop Med Int Health,* 2002, 7: 1068-75.

[53] Leroy EM, Telfer P, Kumulungui B, et al. 'A serological survey of Ebola virus infection in Central African nonhuman primates', *J Infect Dis,* 2004, 190: 1895-9.

[54] Fisher-Hoch SP, Tomori O, Nasidi A, et al. 'Review of cases of nosocomial Lassa fever in Nigeria: the high price of poor medical practice', *BMJ,* 1995, 311: 857-9. p. 857.

[55] Fisher-Hoch SP. 'Lessons from nosocomial viral haemorrhagic fever outbreaks', *Brit Med Bull,* 2005, 73 and 74: 123-37. p. 134.

[56] Ibid. pp. 133-134.

Chapter 9

FAILING TO PROVIDE SAFE HEALTHCARE, 1989-2007

Healthcare involves two parties: those who provide it, and those who receive it. When healthcare is unsafe, both parties have failed. Providers have failed to 'first do no harm.' The public – together with government and civil society organizations – have failed to demand safe care. This chapter discusses the providers' failure, and the next chapter discusses how the public can demand safe care.

Different responses to unexplained HIV infections

Investigations in Russia and Romania, 1988-92

In late 1988, doctors in Elista, Russia, found an HIV-positive child with an HIV-negative mother. Suspecting that the child might have acquired HIV infection as an inpatient at a local hospital in mid-1988, the Ministry of Health tested other children who had been inpatients at the same time. When these tests found more HIV-positive children, the Ministry traced where and when they might have been infected during earlier treatment (see references in Table 9.1). In this way, investigators found the source of the outbreak in a child who had been hospitalized in early 1988. The child's father had received a blood transfusion in Brazzaville, Congo, in 1981, and had subsequently infected the mother, who infected the child.

Extending the investigation to other hospitals, the Ministry of Health found that from May 1988 through August 1989, 13 hospitals in Elista and elsewhere in the region had spread HIV from that one child to more than 260 children. HIV appears to have passed from child to child through intravenous catheters, intramuscular injections, and possibly other equipment and procedures. In addition, 22 mothers acquired HIV from their children, most likely through breastfeeding.

In June 1989, about the time that Russia's Ministry of Health stopped the Elista outbreak, doctors in Bucharest, Romania, unexpectedly found HIV in a hospitalized girl. Testing more inpatient children in the same hospital, doctors found that 12 of 30 were infected. Concerned doctors extended testing to other hospitals, finding more infections. Through mid-1991, tests on more than 29,000 people found almost 1,500 to be infected, 93 percent of whom were children aged 0-3 years (see references to Table 9.1). Only a small minority of their mothers were HIV-positive. Transmission continued into the early 1990s, infecting more than 10,000 children before hospitals and orphanages implemented adequate infection control. One plausible theory to explain the coincident outbreaks in children throughout Romania beginning in the late 1980s is that a locally produced, HIV-contaminated blood product (gamma globulin) infected children in multiple districts, after which HIV spread from child to child through unsterile injections.

Not investigating unexplained HIV infections in Africa, 1984-93

While Russian and Romanian doctors and governments responded to unexplained HIV infections with alarm and investigations, doctors and governments in Africa did not investigate HIV infections in African children with HIV-negative mothers.

For example, at a hospital in Kigali, Rwanda, during 1984-90, Commenges and colleagues found 54 children with AIDS and HIV-negative mothers. They reported that 22 of the 54 had been transfused, but they did not report healthcare risks other than transfusions, and they did not investigate cases by testing other children who had received healthcare at the same clinics and hospitals. Moreover, they showed declining interest to find more unexplained cases: 'The proportion of children [with AIDS] whose mother's serological [HIV] status was investigated decreased over time during the study period.'[1]

Around 1990, WHO's Global Programme on AIDS coordinated studies in the major cities of four African countries – Kigali, Rwanda; Kampala, Uganda; Dar es Salaam, Tanzania; and Lusaka, Zambia – to test inpatient children and their mothers for HIV infection. Combining data from the four cities, WHO reported that 61 (1.1 percent) of 5,593 children aged 6-59 months were HIV-positive with HIV-negative mothers.[2] Only three children had been transfused. WHO's report presented no evidence that infections had come from risks other than blood exposures (such as child sexual abuse, breastfeeding by someone other than the mother, etc.). Incredibly, WHO concluded that 'the risk of...patient-to-patient transmission of HIV among children in health care settings is low.'[3] A similar conclusion would have been unacceptable for WHO as well as for national ministries of health if 1 percent of inpatient children had been found with unexplained HIV infections in almost any country outside Africa.

There is no indication that any of the four governments investigated any of these 61 infections, tracing where children had received medical treatment and testing other children attending those facilities. Neither WHO nor any of the research teams from the four countries has said how many of the 61 unexplained infections were found in each country – information which could have helped people to see and to reduce their risks for HIV infection.

Outbreak investigations continue in countries with concentrated epidemics

The point-counterpoint of investigations in countries with concentrated epidemics but not in countries with generalized epidemics continued into 2007. Some investigations in countries with concentrated epidemics point to risks that may be common in generalized epidemics.

For example, in early 1993, a doctor in New South Wales, Australia, reported to the state government that one of his patients had an unexplained HIV infection, which the doctor suspected had come from invasive procedures at another clinic. The government responded with an investigation, tracing and testing other patients who had visited the suspected clinic on the same day as the patient who triggered the investigation. This investigation found four other patients who were HIV-positive. Four of the five HIV-positive patients had no risk factor other than visiting the clinic. The fifth, an MSM, appears to have been the source of the HIV that infected the others. One hypothesis is that HIV from the source patient got into a multidose vial, from which it was able to reach and infect the other patients.[4] Multidose vials of local anesthetic can be especially dangerous because doctors sometimes re-inject patients who continue to feel pain. If a doctor reuses the same syringe (even with a new needle) to withdraw anesthetic more than once for one patient, this could transfer trace amounts of blood – and pathogens – from the patient to the vial.

The largest documented iatrogenic outbreak occurred in China. Companies buying blood plasma from poor people in rural areas during 1990-95 transmitted HIV to as many as 100,000 or more paid donors (see references in Table 9.1).

Table 9.1: Documented outbreaks of HIV infection from medical procedures*

Country, year of outbreak	Who was infected	Number of cases identified	Search to find all cases?
Mexico, circa 1986[5]	Blood and plasma sellers	281	No
Russia, Elista, 1988-89[6]	Inpatient children	>260	Yes
Romania, circa 1988-1992[7]	Children	~10,000	No
India, Pune, circa 1988[8]	Blood and plasma sellers	97	No
India, Mumbai, circa 1988[9]	Blood and plasma sellers	~172	No
Egypt, 1991 and before[10]	Dialysis patients	82	Yes
Argentina, 1990[11]	Dialysis patients	33	Yes
Columbia, 1992-93[12]	Dialysis patients	13	Yes
Argentina, 1993[13]	Dialysis patients	20	Yes
Egypt, 1993[14]	Dialysis patients	64	Yes
China, 1990-95[15]	Blood and plasma sellers	~100,000	No
Libya, 1997-99[16]	Inpatient and outpatient children	>400	Yes
Kazakhstan, 2006[17]	Children	≥133	Yes
Kyrgyzstan, 2007[18]	Children and adults	≥26†	Ongoing†

* Outbreaks with 10 or more infections, except outbreaks in which most infections come from receipt of blood or blood products.
† In November 2007, this was an ongoing investigation.

In 1998, doctors at a hospital in Benghazi, Libya, discovered HIV-positive children with HIV-negative mothers (see references in Table 9.1). To investigate this outbreak, the government offered HIV tests to children who had been treated at the hospital during 1997-98. The investigation identified more than 400 HIV-positive children. Sequencing of HIV from a large sub-sample of these children found that the infections were related, and that the outbreak likely began from one infection around 1995. Apparently, injections and other invasive procedures passed HIV from child-to-child. As many as 19 mothers appear to have contracted HIV from their children, possibly through breastfeeding.

Very likely many healthcare workers contributed to the outbreak, infecting children through ignorance and carelessness, but with no intention to harm. Unfortunately, the government's investigation went off track to accuse seven foreign healthcare workers – six Bulgarians and a Palestinian – with deliberately infecting the children. Most of the accused did not begin to work at the hospital until years after the outbreak began. Nevertheless, a Libyan court convicted six of the seven for murder, and sentenced them to death. In July 2007, the Libyan government commuted their sentences to life in prison, and transferred them as prisoners to Bulgaria, where the government immediately freed them. They had spent more than eight years in prison.

In July 2006, doctors in southern Kazakhstan discovered children with unexplained HIV infections. This discovery led to an investigation that tested more than 10,000 children and discovered 133 infected children (through late 2007). More than 10 mothers appear to have been infected through breastfeeding. The investigation led to criminal convictions for 21 doctors and officials for actions that contributed to unsafe healthcare.

Lack of investigations continues in Africa and India

Through 2007, journals, newspapers, and other publications have reported hundreds of children in Africa[19] and at least 30 in India[20] with unexplained or nosocomial HIV infections (excluding infections from transfusion of blood or blood products). Such public reports document only a small portion of the unexplained infections that have been recognized. In any city with a generalized epidemic, one can usually find one or more cases by asking around among doctors at major hospitals and counselors at HIV testing centers.

An incomplete investigation in Mumbai, India, in 1997 illustrates dangers to the public when governments do not investigate unexplained infections. In 1996, a Mumbai nursery arranged HIV tests for infants intended for adoption by Danish families. All children tested HIV-negative. In 1997, one child was tested again because of illness – and was found to be HIV-positive. Subsequent testing of all children in the nursery (the report does not say how many) found seven more who were HIV-positive. Sequencing of HIV from six of the eight HIV-positive children found that the viruses were similar, so that the infections were linked. All eight children had received treatment at a Mumbai nursing home in October 1996. Several had received blood or blood products. For five children, the only reported risks were 'intravenous antibiotic treatment and routine immunization.'[21]

A visiting Danish team managed the investigation. A copy of their unpublished report is on file in the office of the Safe Injection Global Network (SIGN) at WHO in Geneva. There is no indication that any government agency extended the investigation to other children who had been treated in the implicated nursing home during 1996, and there is no indication that anyone warned anyone or changed any procedures to protect other children. In 2005, during a visit to Mumbai, I met with government officials and doctors involved in AIDS prevention and in hospital infection control. No one I talked with had heard of the incident or of the Danish investigation.

In 2000, a team at Stellenbosch University in South Africa established a registry of unusual HIV infections among children.[22] Through early 2004, they recorded 16 HIV-positive children with HIV-negative mothers. Two had possible sexual exposures, and one appears to have been infected by close contact with a sibling. All the other 13 had been inpatients prior to their HIV diagnosis.[23] Although the team identified the hospitals where the children might have been infected, the government did not investigate by testing other children who had attended those hospitals. After the Stellenbosch team reported these infections in the *South African Medical Journal*, a subsequent editorial in the *Journal* urged that 'scarce resources should not be devoted to research into the extent of nosocomial transmission of HIV-1.'[24]

A 2004-05 national survey in Uganda tested more than 8,000 children aged 0 to 5 years, and was able to test most of their mothers as well. Approximately 15 percent of the mothers of HIV-positive children tested HIV-negative.[25] A study in south Uganda during 1999-2004 identified 1-3 children who might have contracted HIV from healthcare.[26] In both cases, the analyses noted that most infections were from mother-to-child transmission, and did not report or urge investigations to find the source of the unexplained infections.

Aside from children, studies and surveys have reported hundreds of adults with unexplained infections. These reports are routinely discounted with the suspicion that the men and women had lied about their sexual activities (see Chapter 7). As has happened with children, no African government has investigated any unexplained HIV infection in adults.

AIDS prevention programs pay little attention to healthcare risks

Throughout 1989-2007, officials in WHO's Global Programme on AIDS were aware of widespread and persistent infection control lapses in Africa. In 1991, for example, senior officials noted that in Africa[27]

> ...it has been difficult to ensure proper sterilization procedures because of low equipment-to-patient ratios which make sterilization of equipment between use difficult; lack of sterilization equipment and protective clothing, and irregular power supplies....[A]lthough as few as 60% of needles and 21% of syringes are sterilized in some immunization programmes, these percentages can be increased to over 95% when health staff are retrained and supervision is ensured.

Nevertheless, from the late 1980s, WHO's Global Programme on AIDS shifted attention and money away from patient safety in countries with generalized epidemics. In 1993, the Programme's proposed budgets for HIV prevention in developing countries included only 4-7 percent for blood safety and nothing for infection control.[28] Similarly, the Global Programme did not mention infection control in its own proposed budget for 1994-95.[29]

From end-1995, WHO's Global Programme on AIDS dissolved, passing its work to UNAIDS (the Joint United Nations Programme on HIV/AIDS). UNAIDS is not part of WHO, but is rather a new organization that as of 2006 reported to 10 UN agencies (including WHO, World Bank, UNICEF, and others). UNAIDS was positioned to deal with the AIDS epidemic as an economic and social issue, going beyond the mandates of ministries of health.[30] In this way, the formation of UNAIDS further weakened attention to infection control.

During the 1990s through 2007, international and foreign-supported AIDS programs paid some attention to occupational risks for healthcare workers and to blood transfusions. However, they paid almost no attention to standard precautions to prevent patient-to-patient transmission of HIV. The one major exception – from 2004 – was US aid for injection safety for AIDS prevention.

Not protecting healthcare workers

In the US and in other developed countries, governments in the early 1980s tightened rules and recommendations for healthcare workers to wear gloves and other protective gear and to avoid blood exposures (see Chapter 4). From the late 1980s, hospitals in developed countries began to offer short-term treatment with zidovudine, an antiretroviral drug, to healthcare workers after needlestick accidents. Such treatment – known as post-exposure prophylaxis (PEP) – provides partial protection against HIV infection. Post-exposure prophylaxis became standard in the mid-1990s in rich countries with concentrated epidemics.

AIDS programs in countries with generalized epidemics have allocated funds to protect healthcare workers. However, it has not been enough. Gloves and other protective gear have often been in short supply. Post-exposure prophylaxis was rarely available before 2000, and as of 2007 is still not generally available. In India in 2007, for example, post-exposure prophylaxis was available for government health staff, but not for most private healthcare workers.

In countries with generalized epidemics, HIV infections from occupational blood exposures have only rarely been documented. A worldwide compilation of reported HIV infections among healthcare workers from occupational exposures through 1997 found 94 cases, of which only 4 came from Africa.[31] This is an absurdly low figure, considering that 70 percent of HIV infections have been in Africa, where healthcare workers have much less protective gear than in developed countries.[32] In 2003, a WHO team used information on numbers of needlestick accidents and HIV infections among patients to estimate that occupational exposures infect 1,000 healthcare workers with HIV per year, including more than 800 in Africa and Asia.[33] Continuing high risk for healthcare workers undermines health systems and programs.

Holding back on blood safety

In 1988, WHO's Global Programme on AIDS and the League of Red Cross and Red Crescent Societies established the Global Blood Safety Initiative. In early 1989, after consultations with countries and organizations, the Initiative proposed minimum targets and essential consumables and equipment for blood transfusion services.[34] These proposals fell on deaf ears. A 1989 editorial in the *Lancet* criticized that governments 'have often found it easier to funnel resources into cleaning up the blood supply than into interventions directed at high-risk groups.'[35] In 1991, senior officials in WHO's Global Programme on AIDS recommended that countries should not put too much money into blood safety, so that 'funds are not diverted from higher priority strategies for prevention of HIV sexual transmission.'[36]

Lack of money and support for blood safety has meant that doctors in much of Africa continued to transfuse untested blood. In 1989, for example, a doctor in Burkina Faso wrote to a major medical journal[37]:

> The rainy season is just starting and shortly the wards will be inundated with patients, especially pregnant women and young children, suffering from severe anaemia induced by malaria on top of chronic nutritional anaemias. We have no means of screening blood before transfusion...
>
> We wait for the national anti-AIDS programme to reach our hospital. Meanwhile we work in the dark against a largely unknown enemy, our patients at risk and the AIDS epidemic unchecked.

A 1990 study in Kinshasa found that at least 28 percent of recently transfused blood had not been tested for HIV, the supply of test kits was irregular, many healthcare facilities did not have sterilized instruments on hand, and supposedly sterile instruments were contaminated.[38] A comment on this paper in WHO's *AIDS Technical Bulletin* called the findings 'a horrifying indictment...of the international response to the African AIDS epidemic.'[39]

Even in countries with some of the best blood banking systems in Africa, quality control was a problem. In Uganda, the international community has maintained its own blood supply for expatriates. During a visit to Zimbabwe in the late 1990s, I met a resident foreign health expert who thought about having his arm tattooed, 'Do not transfuse,' so that if he were in a traffic accident and unconscious the medics would see his message.

International AIDS prevention programs that put a low priority on blood safety influenced national programs to do so as well. For example, in the early 1990s, the government of India 'initially requested World Bank support primarily for blood safety,' but 'Following an intensive dialogue with the [World] Bank and WHO' the project was redesigned to emphasize other issues.[40] With the revised design, India proposed to test only 'the majority of blood units.' The government of India did not implement policies to stop HIV transmission through blood transfusions until India's Supreme Court ordered it to do so in 1996.

A 1997 review of blood transfusions in Africa rues that the Global Blood Safety Initiative 'did not receive the financial and other backing commensurate with the proportion of the pandemic fueled by blood transfusion...'[41] Towards the end of the 1990s, WHO formed a Blood Safety Unit to assist member states. This too operated with limited resources. When I visited the unit in 2001, staff presented strategies to ensure safe blood transfusions, but without any budgets or timelines to show that these strategies could be or would be implemented any time soon – or indeed ever.

From 2003, the US Senate directed USAID and CDC to use a portion of money allocated for AIDS prevention in Africa, Asia, and the Caribbean to improve blood safety. During 2004-06, these agencies committed a total of more than $100 million to blood safety in 15 target countries (12 in Africa, and Guyana, Haiti, and Vietnam), although actual spending lagged.[42]

Although most countries in Africa report that all or most blood is tested for HIV, WHO reported in 2006 that less than 12 percent was 'tested for HIV in a quality-assured manner.'[43] As of 2005, WHO estimated that blood transfusions infect 160,000 people worldwide each year,[44] accounting for 5 percent of new HIV infections. This estimate is based on weak data – it is calculated from estimates of the numbers of transfusions and the percentage of transfused blood that is contaminated. In this case, because transfusions are not so common, and because countries with some of the worst HIV epidemics (including especially South Africa) do a pretty good job screening transfused blood, 5 percent may over-estimate the proportion of HIV infections from transfusions.

Because of insufficient attention to sterile procedures, blood donors have also been at risk. Studies in India, China, Mexico, and other countries show that tens of thousands of people have been infected with HIV during blood and plasma donation. In Africa, with rare exceptions, researchers did not ask about blood donation as a risk for HIV infection, even though repeat paid and replacement donors often had higher HIV prevalence than other adults. During hearings on blood safety in Africa in the US Congress in 2006, one witness noted that 'in the United States we take for granted that...the needle is sterile, and that being at the health facility will not threaten our own health,' whereas 'These are all assumptions that do not necessarily apply in Africa.'[45]

Preventing HIV through injections: Too late, too little

Among all public health programs advised and supported by international agencies, the Expanded Programme on Immunization (EPI) was most alert to lapses in infection control. From the end of the 1970s, EPI managers recognized that a large proportion of immunization injections were unsafe. Responses included supplying autoclaves, training healthcare workers and managers, and a search for safer technologies.

In 1987, US Surgeon General Koop asked the US patent office to expedite patent applications for non-reusable injection equipment.[46] In the same year, EPI staff met with inventors and representatives of companies producing syringes to review proposed designs for auto-destruct syringes (that break after one use) and pre-filled disposable syringes that could not be refilled and reused. From these meetings, EPI's experts recognized a number of promising designs, and anticipated 'Volume production...by the end of 1988 for more than one manufacturer.'[47]

For various reasons, including disagreements about the best strategy to ensure safe injections[48] and alleged opposition by at least one syringe producer,[49] the shift to auto-destruct (currently known as autodisable) syringes for immunizations dragged out over several decades. UNICEF's first contract for 80 million syringes asked for delivery to begin in 1992.[50] This was delayed. As of 1996, WHO estimated that only 60 million (6 percent) of 1 billion immunization injections in developing countries used autodisable syringes.[51]

Building support for injection safety

Through the late 1980s, although public health experts were generally aware that injections in Africa and Asia were often unsafe, they had only a vague sense of the size of the problem. From 1989, surveys provided progressively better information about the numbers of injections and the frequency of unsafe practices.

In six African countries during 1989-90, adults reported an average of 1.7 to 2.7 injections per year.[52] A WHO-sponsored study in Uganda in the early 1990s found that 37 percent of households reported a history of an injection-related abscess, and that healthcare facilities often reused equipment without sterilization. One clinic, for example, sterilized its three syringes once each day, but reused them to inject an average of 15 patients per day.[53] A 1997 study of immunization injections in 26 health facilities in Swaziland found that health staff in eight facilities changed needles while reusing syringes, and in two facilities reused disposable syringes and needles.[54]

During 1995-98, WHO surveyed injection practices in 13 African countries. A WHO summary of findings from these surveys concluded:[55]

> ...the study countries have not made any progress with regard to safety over the last 10 years. The high rates of injection-associated abscesses indicate that injection practices are still poor. However, abscesses only represent the tip of the iceberg of AEFIs [adverse events following immunization]. In Africa, where hepatitis B virus (HBV) and the human immunodeficiency virus (HIV) are very prevalent, transmission of bloodborne pathogens from one patient to another...could lead to a much higher burden of initially asymptomatic chronic diseases.

Unsafe injections reflect, in part, lack of knowledge among health care workers about what is required to give a safe injection. For example, 81 percent of doctors surveyed in India[56] in 1992, and 91 percent of healthcare workers surveyed in Ethiopia[57] in 2003-04 thought that an injection was safe if the provider changed the needle but reused the syringe.

During the 1990s, WHO's EPI staff recognized that 'Rapid and substantial progress towards safer injections needs a much broader approach to encompass all types of injections,' not only injections for immunization.[58] EPI found allies for injection safety in WHO's Action Programme on Essential Drugs, USAID, CDC, and elsewhere. In 1994, African ministers of health meeting in Yamoussoukro, Cote d'Ivoire, endorsed a declaration that 95 percent of injections for immunization should use sterile syringes and needles by 1997.[59] However, not everyone associated with immunizations was equally concerned about injection safety. Notably, the strategic plan for 1998-2001 of the Global Programme for Vaccines and Immunization did not mention injection safety among its 12 priorities.[60]

Late progress towards injection safety

In 1999, advocates for injection safety achieved major breakthroughs. In October 1999, the *Bulletin of the World Health Organization* published a landmark paper that reported previously unpublished information from WHO-sponsored surveys of injection practices during 1987-1999. In 10 of 12 African and Asia countries from which data were available (listed by region, but naming only five countries) healthcare workers had reused syringes or needles without sterilization for 50 percent to more than 90 percent of injections.[61] Health officials in WHO and in member governments had kept this information away from populations at risk. By not reporting most of these data according to countries, they continued to do so. A companion paper in the same issue of the *Bulletin* estimated that unsafe injections in developing and transition countries infected 80,000-160,000 people with HIV in a year,[62] which was roughly 2-4 percent of estimated HIV incidence (see Chapter 8).

This accumulated evidence was too much to ignore. In 1999, WHO identified 'immunization safety' as a priority program within the Department of Vaccines and Biologicals, and established a Steering Committee on Immunization Safety to advise the Department. The report of the first meeting of the Steering Committee acknowledges – 25 years after EPI began – that 'up to one-third of immunization injections are not carried out in a way that guarantees sterility.'[63]

In the same year, WHO together with UNICEF and the UN Population Fund set a goal to shift immunization injections to autodisable syringes by the end of 2003.[64] Along with this new policy, WHO along with other organizations established the Safe Injection Global Network (SIGN) as a loose affiliation of public and private organizations. With a small secretariat housed in WHO's offices in Geneva, SIGN worked with public and private organizations to reduce unsafe practices not only for immunizations, but also for curative injections.

SIGN also promoted national assessments of injection practices that progressively improved information about injection numbers and practices. In 2002, a WHO team used information from new studies to estimate that Africans received an average of 2.0-2.2 injections per person per year, of which 17-19 percent reused syringes and/or needles without sterilization.[65] A massive study of injection practices in India during 2002-03 reported an average of 5.8 injections per person per year, of which 23 percent reused unsterile or unreliably sterile syringes and/or needles.[66] Unsafe injections in India were more common in four southern states with relatively high HIV prevalence than in most other states.

During 2002-03, an unpublished review commissioned by UNAIDS along with several articles in medical journals proposed that injections might be responsible for much more than 5 percent of HIV infections (see Chapter 8). WHO and UNAIDS rejected these new estimates. However, the US Senate responded with several hearings,[67] and subsequently pressed the US government to use a portion of the funds allocated for AIDS prevention to promote infection control. During 2004-06, the US provided roughly $2 million per country per year for injection safety in 12 African countries and Guyana, Haiti, and Vietnam (funding varied by country). But the US cut this funding back to about $1 million per country in 2007.

As of 2007, immunization injections are safer, but not safe. UNICEF and other international and foreign aid agencies have shifted immunization support to autodisable syringes. From 2006 India shifted all centrally-funded immunizations to autodisable syringes, and many other – but not all – developing countries have done so as well. However, donors and countries continue to rely on multidose vials containing vaccine for as many as 20 patients, which are a risk to spread bloodborne pathogens. Although there was much left to do, in 2005 WHO disbanded the Steering Committee on Immunization Safety.[68]

Less progress has been achieved with curative injections, which account for more than 90 percent of injections. Autodisable syringes have made few inroads into this market. As of late 2007, only a few governments, including governments of Nigeria, Uganda, and Kerala state in India, promote autodisable syringes for curative injections. Furthermore, autodisable syringes are, at best, only part of the solution for curative injections. People get too many (unnecessary) injections, and reuse cannot be avoided for some specialized injection equipment.

Other invasive procedures: Not enough information

Taken together, other blood exposures in formal and informal healthcare and cosmetic services could well be more important than injections in transmitting HIV and other bloodborne pathogens. Unfortunately, there is only spotty information about the frequency of other common procedures, and about percentages of procedures that are unsafe.

A study of infection control in maternity wards in Free State, South Africa, in 2004 found traces of blood on 11 of 49 instruments that regularly come into contact with mothers' or infants' wounds or mucous membranes, such as forceps, scissors, and staple guns.[69] In dental clinics, the same study found traces of blood on 17 of 69 items such as gloves, drill heads, and forceps. In dental clinics, 'Visible blood was noted on 15 items, 12 of which were immediately used for the next patient without cleaning.'[70]

In India, doctors have been observed to reuse suture needles for eye surgery after soaking in disinfectant or wiping with alcohol (precautions which are not adequate to kill HIV).[71] In Africa and India, saline infusions are popular and common. Recent research on blood exposures in India heard from people in several states that doctors reused needles and tubes without sterilization to give infusions.[72]

In India, men and women reported standing in line for tattoos administered with the same needles and inkpots. With such practices, HIV and other bloodborne pathogens can pass from client to client both on the needles and through the ink.[73]

Beginning in 1999, USAID has sponsored national surveys to assess the ability of public and private health facilities to provide various kinds of health services. Along with other issues, these 'Service Provision Assessments,' examine each facility's capacity to sterilize instruments – equipment, knowledge, and written guidelines – but do not look at actual practices. Through late 2007, survey results are available from five countries with generalized HIV epidemics. In each country, Service Provision Assessments focused on facilities delivering maternal and child healthcare and/or HIV/AIDS testing and care (and in one case, family planning services). Of the five, Rwanda's healthcare facilities were best equipped to sterilize instruments. But even in Rwanda, only 87 percent of facilities had equipment to autoclave, boil, or steam instruments. In Ghana, Guyana, Kenya, and Zambia, surveys during 1999-2005 found that only 55-79 percent of facilities had equipment to sterilize instruments (through autoclaving, high-level chemical disinfection, dry heat, boiling, or steaming).[74]

Miscellaneous studies and a handful of Service Provision Assessments in countries with generalized HIV epidemics provide suggestive evidence that infection control has been unreliable for all invasive procedures, not only for injections. But there is no systematic information on actual practices. As far as I know, no UN agency or other organization involved in health aid and advice has even begun to develop survey instruments to monitor the frequency, safety, and location of all invasive procedures.

Women at risk

Some evidence shows that women receive more invasive healthcare than men. A study of admissions to a mission hospital in northern Uganda during 1992-2004 found 1.8 women admitted for every man in the age range 15-44 years. In that age range, 'delivery and gynaeco-obstetrical conditions' and 'inflammatory diseases of the female pelvis' accounted for more than 40 percent of women's admissions. The study summarized that 'women suffer disproportionately from their reproductive role.'[75]

Antenatal care in African and Asia commonly includes taking venous blood (to test for syphilis) and tetanus vaccinations. Immunization schedules in most African countries prescribe five tetanus vaccinations for women,[76] and two are often given in the several months before delivery.

WHO, UNICEF, and the UN Population Fund estimate that at least 5 percent of births require caesarean sections to protect mother or child.[77] In some African communities, caesarean sections are already common. For example, a study in rural Zimbabwe in 1992-93 reported that 6.3 percent of 831 deliveries were caesarean.[78] Although induced abortions are illegal across most of Africa, they are common. WHO estimated 4.2 million abortions annually (14 per 100 live births) in Africa around the year 2000, and 7.2 million annually (18 per 100 live births) in south-central Asia.[79]

Some birth control methods involve invasive procedures. As of 2005, an estimated, 4.8 percent of married women of reproductive age in Africa (including more than 10 percent in Botswana, Kenya, Lesotho, Madagascar, Malawi, Namibia, South Africa, and Swaziland) used injectable hormones for birth control, most often Depo-Provera injected every three months.[80] Injectable hormones have been rare in India. On the other hand, 34 percent of married women in India and 14 percent in Southern Africa relied on female sterilization for birth control.[81] India's family planning program offers female sterilization (tubal ligations) to poor women in health camps (temporary clinics with visiting doctors). Observers at one health camp reported that the surgical team sterilized 48 women in just over two hours. The time allowed for each surgery appeared too brief to sterilize the instruments.[82]

Vaginal exams can expose women to sexually transmitted pathogens. In India, for example, healthcare staff commonly reuse specula without sterilization. Healthcare staff who use gloves to protect themselves may not sterilize or discard them between patients. Surveys of facilities offering maternal and child healthcare in Ghana, Kenya, and Rwanda during 2001-04 found that sterile gloves were available in only 48-67 percent of facilities.[83] 'Promiscuous' specula and gloves could spread genital herpes and other sexually transmitted disease.

Organizations and initiatives promoting healthcare for women include the UN Population Fund, which started in 1970,[84] and the Safe Motherhood Initiative, which began in 1987.[85] No organization promoting healthcare for women has systematically surveyed and reported infection control practices in women's healthcare in countries with generalized HIV epidemics.

Healthcare for sex workers

Relative to other women, sex workers have more risks to acquire HIV infections not only from sex, but also from blood exposures. Sex workers seek frequent injections to treat and even to prevent sexually transmitted disease. In a 1987 study in Nigeria, most sex workers reported 'injections of antibiotics as prophylaxis against infection.'[86] In Tamil Nadu, India, some sex workers thought they were at low risk for HIV infection because, 'I take injections regularly to prevent diseases.'[87] In Thailand during the early 1990s, brothel owners injected sex workers with Depo-Provera to prevent pregnancies. In Chennai, India, many brothel owners arranged for private doctors to give weekly injections of antibiotics to control sexually transmitted diseases.[88]

UNAIDS, USAID, Gates Foundation, and other donors have funded and/or promoted treating sex workers for sexually transmitted disease as a component in AIDS prevention programs. Because of insufficient attention to infection control, these initiatives could also spread HIV. Healthcare for sex workers, a stigmatized group, is likely no safer than for other adults. The only two studies I have found that looked at infection control practices during healthcare for sex workers surveyed facilities treating sexually transmitted disease in Maharashtra, India.[89] Both studies asked about gloves to protect healthcare staff, but ignored risks to sex workers.

World Alliance for Patient Safety promotes learning from errors

During the UN General Assembly Special Session on HIV/AIDS in 2001, governments committed 'By 2003, [to] implement universal precautions in health-care settings to prevent transmission of HIV infection...'[90] The goal was not achieved by 2003, but the commitment remains.

In formulating strategies to ensure universal precautions in Africa and Asia, it is relevant to consider EPI's experience. During the 1980s and 1990s, EPI provided autoclaves, spare parts, training, and supervision to promote use of sterile syringes and needles. In 1999, EPI determined that all of its aid and efforts for 25 years had not been enough to ensure that syringes and needles were sterilized before being reused. The solution that EPI arrived at – to shift immunization injections to autodisable syringes – should ring alarms among healthcare providers and patients. Sterilization may not be reliable!

Although autodisable syringes reduce equipment reuse for immunizations, and may do so as well for curative injections, sterilizing and reusing equipment cannot reasonably be avoided during deliveries, dental care, surgeries, and other healthcare procedures. At the same time, EPI's experience demonstrates that it is not enough for healthcare managers to train, encourage, and promote sterilization of reused instruments. These activities are all necessary, but they are not enough to ensure that instruments are sterilized.

If healthcare is to be safe, errors must be rare. An efficient way to ensure that errors are rare is to look for them, learn from them, and correct them. WHO began to emphasize this approach in 2004 with the formation of the World Alliance for Patient Safety, which is tasked to advise and assist WHO member countries to improve patient safety. One of the first initiatives of the Alliance was to develop guidelines for 'adverse event reporting and learning systems.' 'Adverse events' are instances in which patients have been harmed, and 'potential adverse events' are mistakes that could harm patients. According to these guidelines, healthcare organizations should ensure that 'reporting is safe for the individuals who report,' that 'reporting leads to a constructive response,' and that reports are analyzed and changes proposed.[91]

The Alliance, with its emphasis on reporting and learning from adverse events, could make an important contribution to infection control for HIV prevention. On the other hand, if it ignores problems, it becomes an obstacle, by implicitly assuring people that all is well, or at least not so bad that change is required. When a guard dog does not bark, people think there is no danger. In its first several years, the Alliance has been a dog that does not bark. Silence on key issues undermines its potential contribution to improve patients' safety.

Investigating adverse events

Through late 2007, at least four countries with concentrated HIV epidemics (see Table 9.1) responded to unexplained HIV infections in children with thorough investigations, testing thousands of possibly exposed children. No country with a generalized HIV epidemic – all of which receive substantial amounts of health aid – has done so.

Some evidence suggests that international agencies and foreign aid programs have discouraged investigations. In 1994, the head of WHO's Global Programme on AIDS and the future head of UNAIDS criticized publicity given to Russia's 1988-89 nosocomial HIV outbreak.[92]

> The media, which has publicized nosocomial outbreaks, has helped to increase public awareness about the dangers of nosocomial transmission. But the short-term benefits of increased public awareness may not always be positive [*sic*]. The current outbreak of diphtheria in Russia...has been blamed in part on publicity surrounding nosocomial HIV transmission in southern Russia and other problems in the health-care system, which are thought to have

discouraged mothers of young children from seeking immunizations from a health-care system that they perceived to be unsafe.

During the Safe Injection Global Network's annual meeting in Nairobi in 2003, a health officer from Burkina Faso asked for help to investigate unexplained HIV infections in children. WHO staff who were attending the meeting sat silent.

Through early 2007, the World Alliance for Patient Safety has said nothing to encourage investigations of unexplained HIV infections – adverse events – in countries with generalized epidemics. There have been many opportunities to do so. For example, the Alliance could have praised the government of Kazakhstan for investigating unexplained infections in children in 2006, and could have recommended Kazakhstan's investigation as an example for African governments. The Alliance has also been silent about mounting numbers of unexplained HIV infections in African adults with no reported sexual risks.

Investigating potential adverse events

In countries where governments and courts enforce standard precautions, reported lapses lead to investigations. For example, when a clinic in California found that a healthcare worker had been reusing equipment to draw blood, the company that operated the clinic fired the worker and tested more than 15,000 people for bloodborne viruses.[93] In contrast, in much of Africa and Asia, government health officials who hear about reuse of unsterile instruments may take steps to change the practice, but they rarely call anyone for tests. For example, when a 2004 study in South Africa reported common reuse of unsterile and even visibly bloody instruments in dental clinics,[94] no one made any effort to find and test patients at risk.

When potential adverse events are common, not all events can be investigated. When they occur in a wide range of formal and informal settings, multiple strategies are required to monitor and to respond. During 2004-07, the Alliance repeated previous WHO estimates about the frequency of unsafe injections,[95] but was silent about the inadequacy of current strategies to identify and to respond to common and even routine reuse of invasive instruments without sterilization in varied settings.

Not warning the public

During the last several decades, in countries with high prevalence of hepatitis B and C and HIV infection, ministries of health have not investigated unexplained infections, and have often withheld findings showing frequent reuse of syringes and needles in health facilities. At the same time, WHO and ministries of health have urged the public to come for immunizations, blood tests, treatment of sexually transmitted disease, and other invasive procedures. In 2003, health experts criticized that public discussion of evidence linking healthcare to HIV could 'undermine confidence in health care and vaccinations globally.'[96]

In effect, healthcare professionals have asserted that they should decide the level of risk that is acceptable for patients in Africa and Asia. This transgresses medical ethics, which enjoin doctors to give patients accurate information about risks, leaving patients to decide how much risk they want to accept. Risk is something that even illiterate people can understand. Farmers deal with uncertainty about the weather. Prostitution may be the oldest profession, but gambling and bookmaking are not far behind. Moreover, not warning the public about dangers with unsterilized instruments disregards the role of an informed public in helping to devise, support, and enforce solutions.

---

[1] Commenges D, Alioum A, Lepage P, et al. 'Estimating the incubation period of paediatric AIDS in Rwanda', *AIDS,* 1992, 6: 1515-20. p. 1517.

[2] Hitimana D, Luo-Mutti C, Madraa B, et al. 'A multicentre matched case control study of possible nosocomial HIV-1 transmission in infants and children in developing countries', *9th Int Conf AIDS,* Berlin 6-11 June 1993. Abstract no. WS-C13-2. Available at:
http://www.aegis.com/aidsline/1993/nov/M93B3075.html (accessed 9 September 2007).

[3] Global Programme on AIDS. *1992-1993 Progress Report, Global Programme on AIDS.* Geneva: WHO, 1993. p. 85.

[4] Chant K, Lowe D, Rubin G, et al. 'Patient-to-patient transmission of HIV in private surgical consulting rooms [letter]', *Lancet,* 1993, 342: 1548-1549; Collignon P. 'Patient-to-patient transmission of HIV [letter]', *Lancet,* 1994, 343: 415; Shields JW. 'Patient-to-patient transmission of HIV [letter]', *Lancet,* 1994, 343: 415.

[5] Avila C, Stetler HC, Sepúlveda J, et al. 'The epidemiology of HIV transmission among paid plasma donors, Mexico City, Mexico', *AIDS*, 1989, 3: 631-3.

[6] Pokrovskii VV, Eramova II, Deulina MO, et al. 'An intrahospital outbreak of HIV infection in Elista [in Russian]', *Zh Microbiol Epidemiol Immunobiol*, 1990, 4: 17-23; Pokrovsky VV. 'Localization of nosocomial outbreak of HIV infection in southern Russia in 1988-89', *8th Int Conf AIDS*, Amsterdam 19-24 July 1992. Abstract no. PoC 4138; Sauhat SR, Kotova EA, Prokopenkova SA, et al. 'Risk factors for HIV transmission in hospital outbreak', *8th Int Conf AIDS*, Amsterdam 19-24 July 1992. Abstract no. PoC 4288.

[7] Patrascu IV, Dumitrescu O. 'The epidemic of human immunodeficiency virus infection in Romanian children', *AIDS Res Hum Retroviruses*, 1993, 9: 99-104; Drucker E, Apetrei C, Heimer R, et al. 'The role of unsterile injections in the HIV pandemic', in Sande MA, Volberding PY, Lange J, et al. *Global HIV/AIDS Medicine*. Philadelphia: Saunders, 2007. pp. 755-67; Apetrei C, Loussert-Ajaka I, Collin G, et al. 'HIV type 1 subtype F sequences in Romanian children and adults', *AIDS Res Hum Retroviruses* 1997; 13: 363-5.

[8] Banerjee K, Rodrigues J, Israel Z, et al. 'Outbreak of HIV seropositivity among commercial plasma donors in Pune, India [letter]', *Lancet*, 1989; ii: 166.

[9] Bhimani GV, Gilada IS. 'HIV prevalence in people with no fixed abode – A study of blood donorship patterns and risk determinants', *8th Int Conf AIDS*, Amsterdam 19-24 July 1992. Abstract MoC00937.

[10] Hassan NF, El Ghorab NM, Abdel Rehim MS, et al. 'HIV infection in renal dialysis patients in Egypt [letter], *AIDS*, 1994, 8: 853.

[11] Dyer E. 'Argentinian doctors accused of spreading AIDS', *BMJ*, 1993; 307: 584.

[12] Velandia M, Fridkin SK, Cardenas V, et al. 'Transmission of HIV in dialysis centre', *Lancet*, 1995, 345: 1417-21.

[13] Dyer E. 'Argentinian doctors accused'.

[14] El Sayed NM, Gomatos PJ, Beck-Sague CM, et al. 'Epidemic of human immunodeficiency virus in renal dialysis centers in Egypt', *J Infect Dis*, 2000, 181: 91-7.

[15] Wu Z, Liu Z, Detels R. 'HIV-1 infection in commercial plasma donors in China [letter]', *Lancet*, 1995, 346: 61-2; Wu Z, Rou K, Detels R. 'Prevalence of HIV infection among former commercial plasma donors in rural eastern China', *Health Policy Plan*, 2001, 16: 41-6; Ministry of Health, China, UNAIDS, WHO. *2005 Update on the HIV/AIDS epidemic and response in China*. Geneva: WHO, 2006.

[16] Visco-Comandini U, Cappiello G, Liuzzi G, et al. 'Monophyletic HIV type 1 CRF02-AG in a nosocomial outbreak in Benghazi, Libya', *AIDS Res Hum Retroviruses*, 2002, 18: 727-32; de Oliviera T, Pybus OG, Rambaut A, et al. 'HIV-1 and HCV sequences from Libyan outbreak', *Nature*, 2006, 444: 836-7.

[17] Dosybiev D. 'HIV infection trial offers little closure', Institute for War and Peace Reporting, 11 July 2007. Available at: http://uqconnect.net/signfiles/Archives/SIGN-POST00405.txt (accessed 9 September 2007); 'Kazakhstan: more HIV-infected children found in southern Kazakhstan', RadioFreeEurope/RadioLiberty, 3 October 2007. Available at: http://uqconnect.net/signfiles/Archives/SIGN-POST00405.txt (accessed 10 October 2007).

[18] Shersen D. 'Kyrgyzstan: Officials grapple with HIV outbreak', EurasiaNet, 30 October 2007. Available at: http://uqconnect.net/signfiles/Archives/SIGN-POST00419.txt (accessed 1 November 2007).

[19] Gisselquist D, Potterat JJ, Brody S. 'HIV transmission during pediatric health care in sub-Saharan Africa: Risks and evidence', *S Afr Med J*, 2004, 94: 109-16.

[20] Singhal T. 'Burden of HIV in India due to unsafe injections and blood transfusions', MSc thesis submitted to University of London, 2002; Correa M, Gisselquist D. *HIV from Blood Exposures in India – An exploratory study*. Colombo: Norwegian Church Aid, 2005.

[21] Christiansen CB, Nielsen C, Machucca R. 'Cluster of HIV-1 infection among children in Indian Hospital in Bombay. Informal report to WHO, September 1998.' Department of Virology, Statens Serum Institut, Copenhagen, Denmark.

[22] van Zyl GU, Cotton MF, van Rensburg EJ. 'Registry: Unusual HIV transmission in children under the age of 10 years', *So Afr Med J*, 2000, 90: 1064-5.

[23] Hiemstra R, Rabie H, Schaaf H, et al. 'Unexplained HIV-1 infection in children – documenting cases and assessing for possible risk factors', *So Afr Med J*, 2004, 94: 188-93.

[24] Farham B. 'Risk of HIV transmission during paediatric health care in sub-Saharan Africa', *So Afr Med J*, 2004, 94: 342-3. p. 343.

[25] ORC Macro. *Uganda HIV/AIDS Sero-Behavioural Survey 2004-05*. Calverton, Maryand: ORC Macro, 2006.

[26] Birao S, Morison LA, Nakiyingi-Miiro J, et al. 'The role of vertical transmission and health care-related factors in HIV infection of children: A community study in rural Uganda', *J Acquir Immune Defic Syndr*, 2007, 44: 222-8.

[27] Heymann DL, Edstrom K. 'Strategies for AIDS prevention and control in sub-Saharan Africa', *AIDS*, 1991, 5 (suppl 1): S197-208. p. S201.

[28] Global Programme on AIDS, WHO. 'The cost of HIV/AIDS prevention strategies in developing countries.' Doc. no. GPA/DIR/93.2. Geneva: WHO, 1993.

[29] Global Programme on AIDS, WHO. 'Proposed Programme Budget 1994-95.' Doc. no. GPA/DIR/93.1. Geneva: WHO, 1993.

[30] Public Broadcasting Service. 'Frontline: The age of AIDS – Interview with Peter Piot.' Posted May 2006. Available at:

http://www.pbs.org/wgbh/pages/frontline/aids/interviews/piot.html (accessed 22 September 2007).

[31] Ippolito G, Puro V, Heptonstall J, et al. 'Occupational human immunodeficiency virus infection in health care workers: worldwide cases through September 1997', *Clin Infect Dis*, 1999, 28: 365-83.

[32] Sagoe-Moses C, Pearson RD, Perry J, et al. 'Risks to health care workers in developing countries', *N Eng J Med*, 2001, 345: 538-41.

[33] Pruss-Ustun A, Rapiti E, Hutin Y. 'Estimation of the global burden of disease attributable to contaminated sharps injuries among health-care workers', *Am J Ind Med*, 2005, 48: 482-90.

[34] Global Blood Safety Initiative. 'Consensus Statement on Accelerated Strategies to Reduce the Risk of Transmission of HIV by Blood Transfusion.' Doc. no. WHO/GPA/INF/89.13, Geneva: WHO, 1989.; Global Blood Safety Initiative. 'Minimum Targets for Blood Transfusion Services.' Doc. no. WHO/GPA/INF/89.14, Geneva: WHO, 1989; Global Blood Safety Initiative. 'Essential Consumables and Equipment for a Blood Transfusion Service.' Doc. no. WHO/GPA/INF/89.15, Geneva: WHO, 1989.

[35] 'AIDS: Prevention, policies, and prostitutes', *Lancet* 1989; i: 1111-13. pp. 1112-13.

[36] Heymann DL, Edstrom K. 'Strategies for HIV prevention'. p. S202.

[37] Flander A. 'HIV infection in Africa [letter]', *BMJ*, 1989, 299: 260.

[38] N'tita I, Mulanga K, Dulat C, et al. 'Risk of transfusion-associated HIV transmission in Kinshasa, Zaire', *AIDS*, 1991, 5: 437-9.

[39] Peter Jones. 'Annotation to abstract of N'tita I, Mulanga K, Dulat C, et al. "Risk of transfusion-associated HIV transmission in Kinshasa, Zaire"', *AIDS*, 1991; 5: 437-9, in: *AIDS Technical Bulletin*, 1991, 4: 174.

[40] World Bank. *Project Performance Assessment Report: India National AIDS Control Project (Credit No. 2350)*, Report No. 26224. Washington DC: World Bank, 2003. pp. 2-3.

[41] Fleming AF. 'HIV and blood transfusion in sub-Saharan Africa 1997', *Transfu Sci*, 18, 167-79. p. 172.

[42] 'Making safe blood available in Africa: Hearing before the Subcomm on Africa, Global Human Rights and International Operations of the House Comm on International Relations.' 109th Cong, 2nd Sess (27 June 2006). Testimony by Ryan C, p. 39. Available at: http://commdocs.house.gov/committees/intlrel/hfa28424.000/hfa28424_0f.htm (accessed 9 September 2007).

[43] Ibid. Testimony by Dinghra, p. 130.

[44] WHO. *Global Patient Safety Challenge 2005-2006*. Geneva: WHO, no date. Available at http://www.who.int/gpsc/background/en/index.html (accessed 9 September 2007).

[45] 'Making safe blood available in Africa: Hearing before the Subcomm on Africa'. Testimony by Green E, p. 101.

[46] Marmor M, Hartsock P. 'Self-destructing (non-reusable) syringes', *Lancet,* 1991, 338: 438-9.

[47] WHO. 'Evaluation of injection technologies', Geneva: WHO, 1987. Doc. no. WHO/EPI/CCIS/87.2. p. 9.

[48] Battersby A, Feilden R, Stoeckel P, et al. 'Strategies for safe injections', *Bull WHO,* 1999, 77: 996-1000.

[49] Holding R, Carlsen W. 'Deadly needles: Lost chance to avert crisis', *San Francisco Chronicle,* 28 October 1998; Holding R, Carlsen W. 'Deadly needles: Epidemic's devastating toll', *San Francisco Chronicle,* 29 October 1998.

[50] Marmor M, Hartsock P. 'Self-destructing (non-reusable) syringes'.

[51] WHO. 'State of the world's vaccines and immunization.' Geneva: WHO, 1996. Doc. no. WHO/GPV/96.04.

[52] Ferry B. 'Risk factors related to HIV transmission: Sexually transmitted diseases, alcohol consumption and medically-related injections', in Cleland J, Ferry B (eds). *Sexual Behaviour and AIDS in the Developing World.* Geneva: WHO, 1995. pp. 193-207.

[53] van Staa A, Hardon A. 'Injection practices in the developing world: a comparative review of field studies in Uganda and Indonesia', Doc. no. WHO/DAP/96.4.

[54] Daly AD, Nxumalo MP, Biellik RJ. 'An assessment of safe injection practices in health facilities in Swaziland', *S Afr Med J,* 2004, 94: 194-7.

[55] Dicko M, Oni A-QO, Ganivet S, et al. 'Safety of immunization injections in Africa: Not simply a problem of logistics', *Bull WHO,* 2000, 78: 163-9. p. 166.

[56] Bollinger RC, Tripathy SP, Quinn TC. 'The human immunodeficiency virus epidemic in India: Current magnitude and future projections', *Medicine,* 1995, 74: 97-106.

[57] W/Gebriel Y. 'Assessment of the safety of injections and related medical practices in health institutions at Sidama Zone, SNNPRS', Thesis for the degree of Master of Public Health, 2004, Addis Ababa University.

[58] WHO. 'Report of the Meeting of Interested Parties of the Global Programme for Vaccines and Immunization.' Doc. no. WHO/GPV/98.08. p. 15. Geneva: WHO, 1998.

[59] WHO. 'State of the world's vaccines'.

[60] Global Programme for Vaccines and Immunization, WHO. 'Strategic Plan 1988-2001.' Doc. no.: WHO/GPV/98.04. Geneva: WHO, 1998.

[61] Simonsen L, Kane A, Lloyd J, et al. 'Unsafe injections in the developing world and transmission of bloodborne pathogens: A review', *Bull WHO,* 1999, 77: 789-800.

[62] Kane A, Lloyd M, Zaffran M, et al. 'Transmission of hepatitis B, hepatitis C and human immunodeficiency viruses through unsafe injections in the developing world: Model-based regional estimates', *Bull WHO*, 1999, 77: 801-7.

[63] WHO. 'Report of the first meeting of the Steering Committee on Immunization Safety, Geneva, 25-26 October 1999.' Doc. no.: WHO/V&B/00.17. Geneva: WHO, 2000.

[64] WHO. 'Safety of injections: WHO-UNICEF-UNFPA joint statement on the use of auto-disable syringes in immunization services.' Doc. no.: WHO/V&B/99.25. Geneva: WHO, 1999.

[65] Hauri AM, Armstrong GL, Hutin YJF. 'The global burden of disease attributable to contaminated injections given in health care settings', *Int J STD AIDS*, 2004, 15: 7-16.

[66] India Clinical Epidemiology Network (IndiaCLEN) Program Evaluation Network (IPEN). *Assessment of Injection Practices in India (2002-03)*. New Delhi: IPEN, 2005.

[67] AIDS Crisis in Africa: Health Care Transmission. Hearing before the Senate Committee on Health Education, Labor and Pensions. 108th Cong, 1st Sess (27 March 2003). Available at: http://help.senate.gov/Hearings/2003_03_27/2003_03_27.html (accessed 3 March 2007); Solutions to the Problem of Health Care Transmission of HIV/AIDS in Africa: Hearing before the Senate Comm on Health Education, Labor and Pensions. 108th Cong, 1st Sess (31 July 2003). Available at: http://help.senate.gov/Hearings/2003_07_31/2003_07_31.html (accessed 3 March 2007).

[68] 'Sixth meeting of the Steering Committee on Immunization Safety', *Wkly Epidemiol Rec*, 2005, 80: 389-96.

[69] Shisana O, Mehtar S, Mosala T, et al. *HIV risk exposure among young children: A study of 2-9 year olds served by public health facilities in the Free State, South Africa.* Cape Town: HSRC Press, 2005.

[70] Mehtar S, Shisana O, Mosala T, et al. 'Infection control practices in public dental care services: findings from one South African Province', *J Hosp Infect,* 2007, 66: 65-70. p. 69.

[71] Kermode M, Holmes W, Langkham B, et al. 'Safer injections, fewer injections: Injection safety in rural north India, *Trop Med Int Health*, 2005, 10: 423-32.

[72] Correa M, Gisselquist D. *HIV from Blood Exposures in India.*

[73] Ibid.; Panda S, Kumar MS, Lokabiraman S, et al. 'Risk factors for HIV infection in injection drug users and evidence for onward transmission of HIV to their sexual partners in Chennai, India', *J Acquir Immune Defic Syndr*, 2005, 39: 9-15.

[74] ORC Macro. *Ghana Service Provision Assessment Survey 2002.* Calverton, Maryland: ORC Macro, 2003; ORC Macro. *Guyana HIV/AIDS Service Provision Assessment Survey 2004;* Calverton, Maryland: ORC Macro, 2005; ORC Macro.

1999 Kenya Service Provision Assessment. Calverton, Maryland, ORC Marco, 2000; ORC Macro. *Kenya Service Provision Assessment Survey 2004: Maternal and Child Health, Family Planning and STIs.* Calverton, Maryland: ORC Macro, 2005; ORC Macro. *Rwanda Service Provision Assessment Survey 2001.* Maryland: ORC Macro, 2003; ORC Macro. *Zambia HIV/AIDS Service Provision Assessment Survey 2005.* Calverton, Maryland: ORC Macro, 2006.

[75] Accorsi S, Fabiani M, Nattabi B, et al. 'Differences in hospital admissions for males and females in northern Uganda in the period 1992-2004: A consideration of gender and sex differences in health care use', *Trans R Soc Trop Med Hygiene,* 2007, 101: 929-38. pp. 933, 935.

[76] 'Expanded Programme on Immunization (EPI): Immunization schedules in the WHO Africa Region, 1995', *Wkly Epidemiol Rec,* 1996, 71: 90-95.

[77] AbouZahr C, Wardlaw T. 'Maternal mortality at the end of a decade: Signs of progress? *Bull WHO* 2001; 79: 561-8.

[78] Nilses C, Nystrom L, Munjanja S, et al. 'Self-reported reproductive outcome and implications in relation to use of care in women in rural Zimbabwe', *Acta Obstet Gynecol Scand,* 2002, 81: 508-15.

[79] Ahman E, Shah I. 'Unsafe abortion: Worldwide estimates for 2000', *Reprod Health Matters,* 2002, 10: 13-17.

[80] Population Division, UN. 'World Contraceptive Use 2005.' New York: UN, no date. Available at: http://www.un.org/esa/population/publications/contraceptive2005/WCU2005.htm (accessed 9 September 2007).

[81] Ibid.

[82] Ramanathan M, Dilip TR, Padmadas SS. 'Quality of care in laparoscopic sterilization camps: observations from Kerala, India', *Reprod Health Matters,* 1995, 3: 84-93.

[83] ORC Macro. *Ghana Service Provision Assessment Survey 2002.* Maryland: ORC Macro, 2003; ORC Macro. *Kenya Service Provision Assessment Survey 2004: Maternal and Child Health, Family Planning and STIs.* Maryland: ORC Macro, 2003; ORC Macro. *Rwanda Service Provision Assessment Survey 2001.* Maryland: ORC Macro, 2002.

[84] Department of Economic and Social Affairs, United Nations (UN) Secretariat. 'Fertility, Contraception and Population Policies.' Doc. no. ESA/P/WP.182. New York: UN, 2003.

[85] Inter-Agency Group for Safe Motherhood. *The Safe Motherhood Action Agenda: Priorities for the next decade.* New York: Family Care International, 1998.

[86] Chikwem JO, Ola TO, Gashau W, et al. 'Impact of health education on prostitutes' awareness and attitudes to acquired immune deficiency syndrome (AIDS)', *Public Health,* 1988, 102: 439-45. p. 442.

[87] AIDS Prevention and Control Project (APAC). 'HIV risk behavior surveillance survey in Tamil Nadu, wave VII', Chennai: APAC, no date. p. 28.

Available at: http://apacvhs.org/Pub_Res_BSS.html (accessed 30 September 2007).

[88] Asthana S, Oostvogels R. 'Community participation in HIV prevention: problems and prospects for community-based strategies among female sex workers in Madras', *Soc Sci Med*, 1996, 43: 133-48.

[89] Avert. *Health Care Provider Survey in Maharashtra*. Maharashtra: Avert, 2001; Avert. *Health Care Provider Survey in Maharastra 2004, Round 2*. Maharashtra: Avert, no date.

[90] UN General Assembly. 'Declaration of Commitment on HIV/AIDS', 2 August 2001. Doc. no. A/Res/S-26/2. New York: UN, 2001.

[91] WHO. *WHO draft guidelines for adverse event reporting and learning systems: From information to action*. Doc. no. WHO/EIP/SPO/QPS/05.3. Geneva: WHO, 2005. p. 49.

[92] Heymann DL, Piot P. 'The laboratory, epidemiology, nosocomial infection and HIV', *AIDS*, 1994; 8: 705-6. p. 705.

[93] Porco TC, Aragon TJ, Fernyak SE, et al. 'Risk of infection from needle reuse at a phlebotomy center', *Am J Pub Health*, 2001, 91: 636-8.

[94] Mehtar S et al. 'Infection control practices'.

[95] World Alliance for Patient Safety, WHO. *Global Patient Safety Challenge: Clean care is safer care*. Geneva: WHO, 2005; World Alliance for Patient Safety, WHO. *Forward Programme 2006-07*. Doc. no WHO/EIP/HDS/PSP/2006.1. Geneva: WHO, 2006; WHO. 'Single Use of Injection Devices', *Patient Safety Solutions*, vol. 1, No 8, 2007. Geneva: WHO: 2007. Available at:
http://www.jcipatientsafety.org/24725/ (accessed 27 October 2007).

[96] Garnett GP, Fraser C. 'Let it be sexual – Selection, aggregation and distortion used to construct a case against sexual transmission', *Int J STD AIDS*, 2003, 14: 782-4. p. 782.

Chapter 10

HOW PEOPLE CAN STOP HIV TRANSMISSION DURING HEALTHCARE

> ...the message that other people's blood is extremely dangerous is not yet appreciated in many developing countries.
>
> – Mark Kane, 1998[1]

Because public health managers in countries with generalized epidemics have failed to stop HIV transmission through common blood exposures in healthcare and cosmetic services, it is up to people who are at risk to protect themselves and to demand safe care and services. This is doable with some proven strategies, although application of these strategies will vary from place to place, and from one person to another.

How to protect yourself: Demand investigations

One of the most important things that people can do to protect themselves is to work together to demand investigations of unexplained HIV infections. Unexplained infections are warnings. If nobody investigates smoke, the house might burn down. When an HIV-positive child has an HIV-negative mother, or a wife is HIV-positive with no sexual partners except an HIV-negative husband, these infections are evidence that some clinic or hospital may be infecting others in the community. If no one investigates – testing to find others who have been infected, and to identify the procedures that were responsible – outbreaks can continue with hundreds or thousands of infections (as in Russia, Romania, and Libya).

Without investigations that can identify dangerous clinics and procedures, trying to stop transmission of HIV through healthcare by advising healthcare workers to be careful is like trying to shoot bats on a moonless night. Most healthcare workers think that what they do is safe enough, even though it may not be. Investigations alert healthcare workers to unexpected dangers. And publicity surrounding investigations alerts the public to demand safe care.

In countries where investigations uncovered hospital-based outbreaks, findings from these investigations guided and motivated changes that stopped nosocomial HIV transmission. In Russia, testing after 1989 discovered no new hospital-based outbreaks, although HIV transmits among IDUs. As of 2005, Romania had a concentrated epidemic with less than 0.1 percent HIV prevalence among adults – one of the lowest rates in Europe.

Investigations do not challenge anyone's confidentiality. Whoever is managing an investigation invites people to come for HIV tests based on their attending specific clinics or hospitals during specified periods. No one is required to go for tests, and test results can be confidential. To be accountable to the public, and to help people in the community assess their risks during healthcare, investigators should report their findings in detail – including the number of infections, the ages of those infected, the hospitals and clinics where they were infected, the procedures that transmitted HIV, and so on. Investigators can report such information without disclosing who was infected.

For families with unexplained HIV infections, investigations not only provide explanations, but also bring assistance. In Libya, for example, the government arranged to treat HIV-positive children. Investigations also protect breast-feeding mothers of HIV-positive children and sexual partners of HIV-positive adults by warning them that they are exposed to HIV.

Mobilizing the media, politicians, and courts to achieve investigations

In Russia, government health officials initiated the investigation. In Romania, doctors took the lead. In Libya, parents of infected children pushed the government to investigate.

Public demands for investigation may have to overcome objections from ministries of health, international agencies, and health aid programs as well as from hospitals and clinics subject to investigation. To do so, people can work together to mobilize support through the media, churches, and other civil society organizations. Politicians and their friends and families go for healthcare, so that politicians share the public's concerns about unsafe care. Thus, central or sub-national governments may order ministries or departments of health to investigate. In some countries, courts may be able to order investigations.

When President Yoweri Museveni of Uganda addressed the first AIDS Congress in East and Central Africa in Kampala in 1991, he noted that 'hundreds of children have become infected through the use of unsterilized syringes' in Eastern Europe, and wondered, 'What is happening in our countries, where facilities are worse!' He illustrated his concern with an anecdote:[2]

> I was told a story the other day of a woman taking her child to the hospital...When she got there, the nurse on duty told her that the child needed an injection, but the woman was worried that the syringe might be unsterilized. The nurse said to her, 'For you, madam, we shall use a disposable syringe, but we don't bother to use them on those other common people.' Now, this kind of attitude is completely at variance with medical ethics...

Museveni acknowledged that healthcare providers in Africa worked 'under very difficult conditions,' but challenged them to deliver safe care.

Given Museveni's awareness of investigations in Europe, and his demand that healthcare workers deliver safe care, it is noteworthy that none of the many unexplained HIV infections that have been reported in Ugandan children has led to an investigation. The public and media have not been alert to demand investigations.

No fault investigations?

The community's interest in promoting investigations of unexplained and possibly nosocomial infections is to find out what happened, so that nosocomial transmission can be stopped. Efforts to prosecute or to sue healthcare staff may motivate legal or other strategies to obstruct investigations. One strategy to facilitate investigations may be to release healthcare managers and providers from liability as long as they cooperate with investigators, so that those who have infected patients through carelessness will not be charged with crimes or face civil suits. South Africa's Truth and Reconciliation Commission, which investigated race-related crimes during the apartheid era, provides a model for no-fault investigations.

In Libya and Kazakhstan, investigations that uncovered nosocomial outbreaks led to criminal charges and convictions against healthcare staff. In Libya, convictions made scapegoats of foreign healthcare workers. In Kazakhstan, courts gave harsh punishments to front-line healthcare staff, but suspended sentences to senior managers. In both cases, many who contributed to the culture of carelessness, including WHO and UNAIDS staff in Geneva, were completely out of the picture.

But what happens to those who have been infected through healthcare errors if a country goes for no-fault investigations? In many countries, governments already provide free antiretrovirals for AIDS patients. Even so, governments, churches, and other private groups should consider offering more support to children and others infected through healthcare errors. Even without immunity protecting healthcare providers from civil suits, it is unlikely that more than a small minority of victims would be able to prove who was responsible and to collect compensation.

How to protect yourself: Ask for POST (patient-observed sterile treatment)

In much of Africa and Asia, efforts to promote standard precautions have not ensured safe healthcare in the formal sector. Furthermore, people receive much of their healthcare and cosmetic services from providers in the informal sector, who are beyond the reach of professional education and regulation. Thus, patients and clients would be well-advised to look out for their own safety in both formal and informal settings. To do so, patients and clients can ask service providers to follow practices that will show that instruments are sterile, and that there is no risk to transmit HIV.

For example, when going for injections, patients can ask to see providers take new disposable syringes and needles from sealed plastic packages, and take what is injected from single-dose vials. An acronym that describes these and other similar practices is POST, for patient-observed sterile treatment.[3] For some procedures, such as drilling and filling a tooth, the POST practices that are required to demonstrate that everything is sterile may be more complicated than for injections. Some POST practices might add cost. On the other hand, costs may be lower for some safer practices, such as oral or no medication instead of an injection.

POST practices have already started

Even though the POST strategy has not been systematically promoted anywhere (and few people use the acronym), patients, clients, and service providers have already adopted a variety of practices that fit this strategy. When I visit countries with generalized epidemics, or talk with people who have lived there, I often ask what people do to protect themselves from blood exposures. Awareness varies, as do strategies. Someone from DRC, for example, reported that people going for haircuts bring their own scissors and razors. In India, all barbers I visited in 2005 had shifted from a cut-throat razor (a specialized knife) to a tool that accepts a half-razor as the cutting edge. Each client brings a new razor, or the barber takes one from his stock of new razors. On the other hand, a mother I spoke with in Botswana in 2004 reported that the barber who shaved her young child's head, and who often nicked heads and drew blood, reused instruments without sterilization on child after child. She had not been aware that this was a danger until we talked about it.

During a visit to Mwanza, Tanzania, in 2000, I found that nurses gave pregnant women a list of items to bring for delivery – including plastic gloves, syringe and needle, and razor blade – to protect both healthcare workers and patients. A study in Uganda in the mid-1990s observed that inpatients bring 'a saucepan, cooking stove and fuel' to the hospital. 'At the surgical ward where most patients are receiving over four injections daily,' their attending family or friends 'would boil the equipment once in the morning and later in the evening.'[4] (Although I do not recommend this strategy if other options are available, it illustrates public awareness of risks and patient initiative to ensure safe care.)

Consumer concern about safety has led to more use of disposable syringes. A study of injection practices in 80 clinics in Vellore, India, in the 1990s found that most of them routinely reused syringes and needles without sterilization, and only one patient brought a disposable syringe for own use.[5] From 1995 to 2005, the number of glass syringes sold in India fell by more than 80 percent, while sales of disposable plastic syringes increased by over 500 percent.[6] In a study of injection practices in Ethiopia in 2002, 48 percent of patients brought new disposable syringes for healthcare workers to use to administer injections.[7]

Surveys of injection practices in Uganda in 1993 found that over 60 percent of households brought their own syringes from home. This did not ensure safety because families did not always sterilize them before reuse.[8] Clinics (presumably) used patients' often unsterile syringes to withdraw vaccines and medicines from multidose vials. In this case, ignorance about HIV's ability to survive in syringes for weeks, and to go from syringes to multidose vials, left people with unrecognized risks.

Consumer concern for safety has already had a big impact in favor of safer practices. However, the impact is uneven. Healthcare consumers could achieve better results with more systematic promotion of POST practices, and by working together to demand safe care.

Options to promote POST practices

In much of Africa and Asia, people access most healthcare as outpatients, and pay for much of their care from their own funds, and this is even more so for the poor than for the rich.[9] Thus, patients can protect themselves during one-on-one contacts with providers by asking them to follow POST practices. However, many people, including especially those who are poor or have less education, can be intimidated by healthcare providers, and may find it difficult to request POST practices.

But there are ways that POST can succeed even if most patients are intimidated. First, in situations where providers feel that they are competing for customers, providers might be worried that they will lose customers if they do not accommodate patients' concerns about safety. Thus, providers may adopt POST practices even if only a small minority of their clients is brave enough to ask.

Second, some providers – such as mission hospitals or public clinics – might adopt POST practices not only to ensure that their own procedures are safe but also as an educational device. For example, providers giving an injection with POST practices could explain to patients what they are doing and why, and they could encourage patients to insist on similar POST practices during future healthcare and cosmetic services from other providers.

Third, patients concerned about safety may be able to work with unions, churches, newspapers, private radio shows, local councils, and other civil society organizations to promote POST. This is important, because some organizations that provide healthcare might oppose educating patients to recognize dangerous practices. A church, for example, could organize meetings between members and local healthcare providers. In Thailand in the early 1990s, Empower, a union of sex workers, warned sex workers about risks from unsafe injections. Companies and unions that arrange healthcare or health insurance for workers have an interest not only to protect workers from nosocomial infections, but also to avoid having to pay for AIDS care. Organizations that promote POST could prepare posters illustrating POST practices for injections, tattoos, etc., for service providers to display in their waiting rooms.

Why has the public not demanded safe healthcare?

Not enough HIV testing

Through 2001, not more than about 5 percent of Africans who were HIV-positive were aware of their infections (see Chapter 7). Because HIV prevention messages focused on sex, people without high-risk sexual behaviors would have been less likely to seek tests and to discover their HIV infections. Limited HIV testing thus contributed to public ignorance of unexplained and possibly nosocomial infections.

People are not aware of risks

Because people have been misinformed, they do not know how easy it is to acquire HIV infections from trace amounts of contaminated blood on instruments reused without sterilization. Only 59 percent of senior secondary students in a 1996 survey in Nigeria identified sharing syringes and needles as a risk to transmit HIV.[10] In other recent surveys, 28 percent of South African military recruits did not know that sharing injection equipment was a risk for HIV infection,[11] and only 48 percent of slum residents in Delhi were aware that HIV could be transmitted through unclean syringes.[12] In India, sex workers interviewed in 2005 reported standing in line for tattoos, given without changing or cleaning needles or inkpots between clients.[13] The women thought that was safe, because they believed that HIV survived only seconds outside the body.

People are not afraid of nosocomial outbreaks

Few people in countries with generalized epidemics are aware of the large hospital-based outbreaks of HIV infection among children caused by reused instruments in Russia, Romania, and other countries. Even fewer see those outbreaks as relevant to their communities.

In Africa and India, people sometimes hear about one or more non-vertical and non-sexual HIV infections in children or adults. When such infections can be traced to blood transfusions, public attention sometimes brings changes to make transfusions safer. For example, in Nigeria in 2006, after newspapers picked up the story of an infant infected from transfused blood, the governor of the state fired the head of the hospital that transfused the blood.[14]

However, when an unexplained infection cannot be traced to a transfusion, media and public attention has not pushed governments to investigate to find the extent of the problem and to guide corrective actions. This lack of urgency reflects lack of awareness that one infection might be the tip of an iceberg. One exception illustrates the point. In 2003, *The Sowetan*, a South African newspaper, reported an HIV-negative mother with an HIV-positive child who had never received a blood transfusion.[15] The case was treated as an isolated incident. Neither the media nor the public demanded tests for other children who had attended suspected health facilities, and there was no such investigation.

Why the public might soon demand safe healthcare

More HIV tests

From 2001, two developments brought a major increase in HIV testing in countries with generalized epidemics. The first was the extension of programs to prevent mother-to-child (vertical) transmission by giving antiretroviral drugs to HIV-positive pregnant women and to their babies. In 2001 the UN General Assembly Special Session on HIV/AIDS set goals to reach 80 percent of pregnant women with HIV testing by 2010, and to reduce mother-to-child transmission by 50 percent.[16] In 2001, only about 1 percent of pregnant women in Africa received counseling to prevent mother-to-child transmission. By

2005, an estimated 11 percent of HIV-positive pregnant women received antiretroviral drugs to block mother-to-child transmission.[17]

The second development was the commitment by WHO, donors, and member governments to deliver antiretroviral drugs to all people with AIDS in low- and middle-income countries. In 2003, the WHO established the 3 by 5 program – to put 3 million people in low- and middle-income countries on antiretroviral treatment by 2005. From 2001 to mid-2006, the estimated proportion of Africans with HIV infection and severely weakened immune systems that was taking antiretroviral drugs increased from 1 percent to 28 percent, reaching an estimated 1.3 million people.[18]

These two programs broke the logjam on HIV testing. Whereas most AIDS experts during the 1990s showed little interest in extending testing in countries with generalized epidemics, more and more AIDS experts after 2001 agreed that testing was central to HIV prevention. In 2003, Kevin De Cock, who later became the head of WHO's HIV/AIDS Department, argued that 'universal voluntary knowledge of HIV serostatus should be a prevention goal and that facilitation of HIV testing is central to responding to the epidemic in Africa.'[19] In 2004, health facilities in Botswana began to administer HIV tests routinely to all people who sought healthcare, giving them the option to refuse. In the same year, WHO and UNAIDS endorsed routine testing. Through 2007, routine testing – often called opt-out or provider-initiated testing – spread to other countries in Africa, where it has been adopted in selected facilities.[20]

By 2003-06, national surveys in some African countries found that more than 20 percent of HIV-positive adults had been tested and were aware of their infections, showing a large increase over the situation just a few years earlier. With donors and governments promoting tests, the percentage of HIV-positive people in generalized epidemics who know they are infected is likely to continue to show large increases over the next 3-5 years.

Women on the front lines

Making HIV tests a routine part of antenatal care puts women on the front lines to face HIV-related stigma. Millions of women in Africa and India will soon learn during antenatal care that they are HIV-positive. Women who know they are infected can protect their newborn children and can seek treatment for themselves. However, discovering their infections can also create problems for women. Based on information from recent surveys (Chapter 7), more than half their husbands will be HIV-negative. To protect women from stigma, it is crucial that women's groups, churches, and other organizations do what they can to educate the public that an HIV-infection is not a reliable sign of sexual behavior. This could help women who test HIV-positive to retain the trust, love, and support of their families and friends.

Awareness to action?

With more testing, and especially with routine or opt-out testing during healthcare, many people who know that they had no sexual risks for HIV infection will find they are HIV-positive. More HIV-negative mothers will learn that a child is HIV-positive. This will increase the possibility for a breakthrough in public awareness of the existence – and frequency – of unexplained infections.

When the public is alert to risks in blood exposures, they can find ways – talking to reporters, challenging politicians, going to court, whatever it takes – to demand investigations of unexplained HIV infections, and to ensure that healthcare managers and providers respect demands for safe care. Once healthcare personnel are motivated – by public accountability – technical and organizational changes required within the healthcare system to ensure that healthcare does not transmit HIV will fall into place. All parts of this solution, including information about risks, outrage, accountability, and healthcare system response are local.

Will public demand for safe healthcare stop generalized HIV epidemics?

Vaccines may eventually protect people from HIV infection. Circumcision and microbicides may slow sexual transmission. However, these strategies are either years away and/or do not protect people from HIV transmission through blood exposures. If public demands for investigations and safe practices can stop HIV transmission through healthcare and cosmetic services, many HIV infections will be prevented. How many? No one knows, but it may be enough to stop and to shrink generalized epidemics years before vaccines become available. And if methods to prevent sexual transmission of HIV can be improved, so much the better.

Insofar as the response to HIV leads to more reliable sterilization of reused instruments in healthcare and cosmetic services, the gains in health go far beyond HIV. Hepatitis B and C viruses infect many more people than does HIV. Ebola and other viral hemorrhagic fevers are a continuous threat. But beyond these, other lesser-known and unknown pathogens spread through reused, unsterilized instruments.

Who will explain generalized HIV epidemics?

In several countries in Southern Africa, the chance that an average woman will acquire an HIV infection at some time in her life is well over 50 percent. In many other countries and cities in Southern and East Africa, women's lifetime risk for HIV infection exceeds 25 percent. If a similar disaster were occurring in North America or Europe, the public would demand that their government do whatever is necessary to understand the disaster and to stop it. This has not happened in Africa.

The investigations and research that are required to understand how HIV transmits so much more readily in some countries than in others are standard and easily doable – tracing infections to their sources, to specific sexual partners and to particular clinics, hospitals, or blood exposures. The primary obstacle to doing so appears to have been conflict of interest on the part of healthcare professionals – researchers, managers, and providers – who have not wanted to find HIV transmission through healthcare.

While it is discouraging that international agencies and foreign-funded health aid programs have not promoted or supported the investigations and research that are required to explain generalized HIV epidemics, it is probably best to simply accept it is so, and to get on with the task. Foreign experts and their families are not the ones dying from the epidemic. They carry their own syringes to Africa, and they avoid healthcare they know is not reliably safe.

When a car is heading into a crowd, the people who are in front of the car are the ones at risk, and they are the ones who have to move. By the same logic, it is up to people in countries with generalized epidemics to demand that their governments arrange the investigations and research required to understand and to stop their countries' epidemics.

Investigating and tracing HIV infections to sexual partners and blood exposures could be expected to give a good indication about what is happening within 6-12 months. Such research is likely to lead to one of two findings. One possible finding is that blood exposures account for much of the difference between generalized vs. concentrated HIV epidemics. That would 'solve' generalized epidemics.

The other possible finding is that blood exposures account for some infections, but not enough to explain the difference between generalized and concentrated epidemics. In this case as well, the proposed investigations can be expected to show what drives generalized epidemics. Some experts suppose that men and women with new HIV infections are highly infectious, and account for most heterosexual transmission. Is it so? Others suppose that young women are acutely susceptible to HIV infection during first coitus. Is it so? The verisimilitude of these and other hypotheses could be determined in a matter of months by tracing infections to their sources. Better late then never.

Better understanding of the modes of HIV transmission in countries with generalized epidemics will allow people to protect themselves more effectively from HIV infection. Better information will also guide public health managers to address the most important risks with more focused programs that could slash HIV transmission. In effect, public health experts would be able to draw a red line around the epidemic – to say with confidence that this is how big it will be, and we can control it. That would allow governments and aid programs finally to cap budgets and attention to HIV, and to turn again to other issues.

---

[1] Kane M. 'Unsafe injections', *Bull WHO*, 1998, 76: 99-100.

[2] Museveni YK. *What is Africa's Problem*. Minneapolis: University of Minnesota Press, 2000. pp. 254-5.

[3] Gisselquist D, Friedman E, Potterat JJ, et al. 'Four policies to reduce HIV transmission through unsterile health care', *Int J STD AIDS*, 2003, 14: 717-22.

[4] Birungi H. 'Injections and self-help: Risk and trust in Ugandan health care', *Soc Sci Med*, 1998, 47: 1455-62. p. 1461.

[5] Lakshman M, Nichter M. 'Contamination of medicine injection paraphernalia used by registered medical practitioners in south India: An ethnographic study', *Soc Sci Med*, 2000, 51: 11-28.

[6] Personal communication from Pardeep Sareen, Hindustan Syringes and Medical Devices, 30 December 2005.

[7] Priddy F, Tesfaye F, Mengistu Y, et al. 'Potential for medical transmission of HIV in Ethiopia', *AIDS*, 2005, 19: 348-50.

[8] van Staa A, Hardon A. 'Injection practices in the developing world: A comparative review of field studies in Uganda and Indonesia'. Geneva: WHO, 1996. Doc. no. WHO/DAP/96.4.

[9] Berman P. 'Organization of ambulatory care provision: A critical determinant of health system performance in developing countries', *Bull WHO*, 2000, 78: 791-802.

[10] Fawole OI, Asuzu MC, Oduntan SO. 'Survey of knowledge, attitudes and sexual practices relating to HIV infection/AIDS among Nigerian secondary school students', *Afr J Reprod Health*, 1999, 3 (2): 15-24.

[11] van der Ryst E, Joubert G, Steyn F, et al. 'HIV/AIDS-related knowledge, attitudes and practices among South African military recruits', *S Afr Med J*, 2001, 91: 587-91.

[12] Misra P, Goswami A, Pandav CS. 'Injection safety awareness and knowledge among slum population', *Ind J Community*, 2003, 28(3). Available at: http://www.indmedica.com/journals.php?journalid=7&issueid=55&articleid=67 7&action=article (accessed 13 January 2007).

[13] Correa M, Gisselquist D. *HIV from Blood Exposures in India – An exploratory study*. Colombo: Norwegian Church Aid, 2005.

[14] Anaele A. 'Lagos University Teaching Hospital HIV baby abandoned in ward', *Daily Sun* (Lagos), 27 August 2006. Available at: http://uqconnect.net/signfiles/Archives/SIGN-POST00363.txt (accessed 12 September 2007); 'Lagos Nigeria: Crackdown on dodgy blood banks', *IRIN*, 28 July 2006. Available at: http://uqconnect.net/signfiles/Archives/SIGN-POST00359.txt (accessed 12 September 2007).

[15] Mabena K. 'Mystery over HIV baby', *The Sowetan*, 8 January 2003.

[16] UN General Assembly. 'Declaration of Commitment on HIV/AIDS, 2 August 2001.' New York: UN, 2001. Doc. no. A/Res/S-26/2.

[17] WHO. *Towards Universal Access: scaling up priority HIV/AIDS interventions in the health sector, progress report April 2007*. Geneva: WHO, 2007.

[18] WHO. *The Health Sector Response to HIV/AIDS: Coverage of Selected Services in 2001: Preliminary Assessment*. Geneva: WHO, 2002; WHO. *Towards Universal Access*.

[19] De Cock KM, Marum E, Mbori-Ngacha D. 'A serostatus-based approach to HIV/AIDS prevention and care in Africa', *Lancet*, 2003, 362: 1847-9. p. 1847.

[20] WHO. *Guidance on provider-initiated HIV testing in health facilities.* Geneva: WHO, 2007.

Statistical Annex

For all countries with generalized epidemics, the first section of this Annex presents selected information on HIV prevalence and numbers of infections. The second section provides references to recent national surveys, and identifies these surveys as the sources for tables in Chapters 6 and 7. The third section provides a map of Africa.

HIV prevalence and trends in countries with generalized epidemics

HIV prevalence and infections, 2005-06

The two columns on the right in Annex Table 1 present estimates of HIV prevalence in adults aged 15-49 years and total infections in 2005 for all countries with generalized epidemics. With some adjustments, estimates are from: UNAIDS. *Report on the global AIDS epidemic 2006* (Geneva: UNAIDS, 2006).

Most adjustments are based on data from national surveys. During 2001-07, more than 30 countries with generalized epidemics conducted national surveys of HIV prevalence (see second section of this Annex). For many of these countries, rates of HIV prevalence from surveys are much lower than UNAIDS' 2005 estimates. In such cases, Annex Table 1 reports HIV prevalence from surveys and uses this statistic to adjust UNAIDS' estimated number of infections (the table identifies these survey-based numbers with stars). For example, UNAIDS estimated that 18.8 percent of South African adults were HIV-positive, whereas a national survey in 2005 found 16.2 percent HIV prevalence. From the survey, the table reports 16 percent prevalence for South Africa, and uses that figure to adjust UNAIDS' estimate of 5.5 million infections to 4.7 million [= {16.2/18.8} x 5.5 million].

Other adjustments are based on new estimates in UNAIDS' *AIDS epidemic update December 2007* (Geneva: UNAIDS, 2007). In this publication, UNAIDS cut its estimates of HIV prevalence by 20 percent for Eritrea, the Gambia, Guinea-Bissau, Mozambique, Namibia, Nigeria, Somalia, and Sudan. In addition, UNAIDS cut estimated prevalence in Angola from 3.7 percent to 2.5 percent, and in Madagascar from 0.5 percent to 0.2 percent. Annex Table 1 reports these new estimates for HIV prevalence and adjusts estimated numbers of HIV infections (the table identifies these adjusted estimates with crosses).

With these adjustments, estimated HIV prevalence in Africa falls to 21 million, about 3 million below UNAIDS' initial estimate for 2005.

Trends in HIV prevalence, 1989-2007

To show trends in HIV prevalence over time, Annex Table 1 reports HIV prevalence among women attending urban antenatal clinics. For most countries, the table shows medians among clinics in 'major urban areas' from UNAIDS and WHO's *Epidemiological Fact Sheets on HIV/AIDS and Sexually Transmitted Infections* for various countries and years. The current versions of these *Fact Sheets* are available at http://www.who.int/globalatlas/default.asp. For India, the table shows the medians or means for all sentinel antenatal clinics in each state as reported by India's National AIDS Control Organization (see http://nacoonline.org).

The table shows medians for successive 2-year periods. When medians are available for both years, the table shows the median based on the most clinics, or the median for the earlier year if both years report data from the same number of clinics.

Annex Table 1: HIV prevalence and trends in countries with generalized epidemics, 1989-2006

Region, country (2006 population in millions)	Median HIV prevalence (%), urban antenatal clinics									Adult HIV prevalence in 2005 (%) (year of survey)	HIV infections in 2005 (1,000s)
	'89-'90	'91-'92	'93-'94	'95-'96	'97-'98	'99-'00	'01-'02	'03-'04	'05-'06		
All generalized epidemics, of which:											25,000
Africa											21,000
West Africa											3,800
Benin (8.4)	0.5	0.6	1	2.4	4.3	4	2.3			1.2 (2006)*	58*
Burkina Faso (13)	4.9	7.8		9.6	7.4	7.3	5.3	4		1.8 (2003)*	140*
Cote d'Ivoire (16)	8.4	12	10	14	13	11	6	9.8		4.7 (2005)*	500*
Gambia (1.5)	0.1		0.6		1					1.9†	16†
Ghana (22)	0.7	2.9	1.7	1.3	2.5	2.2	4.1	3.9	2.7	2.2 (2003)*	310*
Guinea (8.2)	1.1		1.2			5	4.1			1.5 (2005)	85
Guinea-Bissau (1.6)	0.2	0.2	1.2	2.7	2.5	4.8				3.0†	26†
Liberia (3.1)		3.7	4							1.5 (2006-07)*	25*
Mali (14)			4.4		2.5	3	3.4	3	4	1.3 (2006)*	100*
Mauritania (3.1)			0.5							0.7	12
Niger (14)		0.8	1.3	0.6		1.8				0.7 (2006)*	50*
Nigeria (132)	1	0.7	4	1		4.5	4.2	4.3		3.1†	2,300†
Senegal (12)	0	0.3	0	1	0.3	0.9	0.8	1.7		0.7 (2005)*	47*
Sierra Leone (4.6)	0.8	1.9	3.1	5.4						1.6 (2005)	48
Togo (6.1)		17		6	6.8		7.9	7.1		3.2	110
Central Africa											2,200
Angola (13)		0.7		1.2	3.8	3.4	8.6	3.8		2.5†	220†
Cameroon (16)	0.8	1.8	3	4.5		12	7			5.4 (2004)	510
Central African Republic (3.8)	8	-	9.3	12	13		15			6.2 (2006)*	140*
Chad (9.7)				2.4		6.2	7.5	5		3.5 (2005)	180
Congo (4.0)	6.8	8.3	7.8	5.2	5.8	10	4		4.4	4.2†	100†
Democratic Republic of Congo (6)	4.7	5.8	5.8	3.2	3	4.1	2.7	4		3.2	1,000
Equatorial Guinea (0.5)				0.7	1.5					3.2 (2004)	9
Gabon (1.4)		1.3	2.3	4			6	8.2		7.9	60

Annex Table 1, continued: HIV prevalence and trends in countries with generalized epidemics, 1989-2006

Region, country (2006 population in millions)	Median HIV prevalence (%), urban antenatal clinics									Adult HIV prevalence in 2005 (%) (year of survey)	HIV infections in 2005 (1,000s)
	'89-'90	'91-'92	'93-'94	'95-'96	'97-'98	'99-'00	'01-'02	'03-'04	'05-'06		
East Africa											5,000
Burundi (7.5)		13	23	28	18	16	16	13		3.3 (2002)	150
Djibouti (0.8)		0.5	4				2.5			3.1	15
Eritrea (4.4)							2.5	3.6		1.9†	47†
Ethiopia (67)	5.1	11	20	19	17	15	16	12		1.6 (2005)*	600*
Kenya (31)	8.9	14	17	17	17	15	14	12		6.1 (2002)	1,300
Somalia (9.1)					0			0.9	1	0.7†	35†
Rwanda (8.1)	27	27		23	19	13	13	13		3.0 (2005)*	190*
Sudan (36)				4.5	0.5			0.3		1.3†	280†
Tanzania (38)	8.9	9.7	15	12	14	15	12	10		6.5 (2003)	1,400
Uganda (24)	27	27	24	19	15	11	11			6.7 (2004-05)	1,000
Southern Africa											10,400
Botswana (1.8)	6	19	28	38	43	44	45	47		24 (2004)	270
Lesotho (1.8)		5.5	6.1	21		42		35		23 (2005)	270
Madagascar (19)	0	0	0	0				0.3		0.2†	20†
Malawi (12)	17	22	21	23	25	25	20	18		12 (2004)*	800*
Mozambique (18)	0.6	1.2	2.7	5.8	11	14	15	21		13†	1,400†
Namibia (1.9)		4.2	6.8	16	26	30	26	16		16†	180†
South Africa (44)	0.6	0.9	3	12	15	21	26	27		16 (2005)*	4,700*
Swaziland (1.0)	-	4.3	22	19	30	32	37	40		26 (2006-07)*	170*
Zambia (11)	25	27	28	26	27	32	27	26		16 (2001-02)	1,100
Zimbabwe (13)	19	28	26	31	30	31	31	20		18 (2005-06)*	1,500*
Caribbean											300
Dominican Republic (8.9)		0.9	1.2	2	1.9	1.2	1.8			1.0 (2002)	66
Haiti (8.5)	7.1		8.4	10		3.8		2		2.2 (2005-06)*	100*
Honduras (7.2)	3.4	3.6	1.4	4.1	1.4	2.9				1.5	63
7 countries‡ (6)										1.5-3.3	82

Annex Table 1, continued: HIV prevalence and trends in countries with generalized epidemics, 1989-2006

Region, country (2006 population in millions)	Median HIV prevalence (%), urban antenatal clinics									Adult HIV prevalence in 2005 (%) (year of survey)	HIV infections in 2005 (1,000s)
	'89-'90	'91-'92	'93-'94	'95-'96	'97-'98	'99-'00	'01-'02	'03-'04	'05-'06		
Asia and Oceania											3,500
Cambodia (14)	0	-	3	0.8	4.9	3.6	5			0.6 (2005)*	50*
India (1,103), of which:										0.36 (2005-06)†	2,500†
Andhra Pradesh (76)				2.3	2.0	1.3	2.3	2.0		0.97 (2005-06)	
Karnataka (53)				1.8	1.7	1.8	1.3	1.3		0.69 (2005-06)	
Maharash-tra (81)				2.0	1.1	1.3	1.3	1.3		0.62 (2005-06)	
Tamil Nadu (62)				1.0	1.0	0.9	0.5	0.5		0.34 (2005-06)	
Manipur, Mizoram, Nagaland (5)				0.5-0.8	0.4-1.4	1.1-1.5	1.3-1.5	0.9-1.6			
Myanmar (51)		0	0	0.8	0.7	1.8			1.3		360
Papua New Guinea (5.9)			0	0.1	0.3	0.3	0.8	1.1		1.8	60
Thailand (64)	0.2	0.6	1.9	1.9	1.3	2.3	1.6	1.1		1.4	580

* For these countries, the table uses HIV prevalence from national surveys to adjust UNAIDS' estimated number of infections.

† For these countries, the table adjusts UNAIDS' 2005 estimates with information from UNAIDS' *AIDS epidemic update December 2007*.

‡ Bahamas, Barbados, Belize, Guyana, Jamaica, Suriname, and Trinidad and Tobago.

Sources for population: UNAIDS. *Report on the global AIDS epidemic 2006*. Geneva: UNAIDS, 2006. For Indian states, population is for 2001 from Wikipedia.

Sources for other columns: See text.

National surveys of HIV infection, 2001-07

More than 25 countries with generalized epidemics have arranged well-designed two-stage random sample surveys. In most cases, the ministry of health supervises the survey and publishes the results. These surveys provide the information about HIV prevalence according to sex, urban and rural residence, education, and socio-economic status that has been presented in Tables 6.2-6.6. These surveys are also the source for information on HIV prevalence in men and women reporting 0-1 sexual partners in the past year (Table 7.1), in virgins (Table 7.3), in circumcised and uncircumcised men (Table 7.4), in women according to age (Figure 7.1), and in couples (Table 7.5).

Annex Table 2a: Sources for national surveys, 2001-07 (surveys for which results are available from ORC Macro, Calverton, Maryland, at http://www.measuredhs.com/countries/start.cfm)

Country	Reference
Burkina Faso	*Burkina Faso Enquete Demographique et de Sante 2003*
Cambodia	*Cambodia Demographic and Health Survey 2005*
Cameroon	*Cameroun Enquete Demographique et de Sante 2004*
Cote d'Ivoire	*Cote d'Ivoire Enquete sur les Indicateurs du SIDA 2005*
Dominican Republic	*Republica Dominicana Encuesta Demografica y de Salud 2002*
Ethiopia	*Ethiopia Demographic and Health Survey 2005*
Ghana	*Ghana Demographic and Health Survey 2003*
Guinea	*Guinee Enquete Demographique et de Sante 2005*
Haiti	*Haiti Enquete Mortalite, Morbidite et Utilisation des Services 2005-2006*
Kenya	*Kenya Demographic and Health Survey 2003*
Lesotho	*Lesotho Demographic and Health Survey 2004*
Malawi	*Malawi Demographic and Health Survey 2004*
Mali	*Enquete Demographique et de Sante Mali 2001*
Niger	*Niger Enquete Demographique et de Sante et a Indicateurs Multiples 2006*
Rwanda	*Rwanda Demographic and Health Survey 2005*
Senegal	*Enquete Demographique et de Sante Senegal 2005*
Tanzania	*Tanzania HIV/AIDS Indicator Survey 2003-04*
Uganda	*Uganda HIV/AIDS Sero-Behavioural Survey 2004-05*
Zambia	*Zambia Demographic and Health Survey 2001-2002*
Zimbabwe	*Zimbabwe Demographic and Health Survey 2005-06*

Annex Table 2b: Sources for national surveys, 2001-07 (surveys recently completed or underway as of late 2007, for which ORC Macro is expected to publish the reports in 2008-09, making them available at: http://www.measuredhs.com/countries/start.cfm)

Country	Reference
Benin	2006 survey. Adult HIV prevalence reported in: UNAIDS. *AIDS epidemic update December 2007*. Geneva: UNAIDS, 2007.
DRC	2007 survey. Results not yet available.
India	2005-06 survey. Results reported in: International Institute for Population Sciences (IIPS), ORC Macro. *National Family Health Survey (NFHS-3), 2005-06: India*: Vol 1. Mumbai: IIPS, 2006. Available at: http://www.nfhsindia.org/volume_1.html (accessed 18 October 2007).
Liberia	2006-07 survey. Some results reported in: Liberia: HIV rates lower than feared. IRIN, 2007. Available at: http://www.irinnews.org/Report.aspx?ReportId=73962 (accessed 24 September 2007).
Mali	2006 survey. Adult HIV prevalence reported in: UNAIDS. *AIDS epidemic update December 2007*. Geneva: UNAIDS, 2007.
Swaziland	2006-07 survey. Some results reported in: Swaziland: new HIV figures reveal extent of epidemic. IRIN, 2007. Available at: http://www.irinnews.org/Report.aspx?ReportId=72999 (accessed 24 September 2007).

Annex Table 2c: Sources for national surveys, 2001-07 (other surveys for which adult HIV prevalence is available from: UNAIDS. *AIDS epidemic update December 2007*. Geneva: UNAIDS, 2007)

Country	Reference
Botswana	2004 survey. Central Statistics Office (CSO). *Botswana AIDS Impact Survey II: Popular Report*. Gbarone: CSO, no date.
Burundi	2002 survey. Ministere de la Sante Publique du Burundi. *Enquete National de Seroprevalence de l'Infection par le VIH au Burundi*. Bujumbura: 2002.
CAR	2006 survey. Adult HIV prevalence reported in: UNAIDS. *AIDS epidemic update December 2007*. Geneva: UNAIDS, 2007.
Chad	2005 survey. Institut National de la Statistique, des Etudes economiques et demographiques et Programme national de Lutte Contre le Sida. *Rapport de l'enquete natioale de seroprevalence du VIH/SIDA au Tchad 2005*. N'Djamena: 2006.

Equatorial Guinea	2004 survey. Programa Nacional de Lucha contea el Sida, Proyecto Centro de Referencia para el control d endemoias en Guinea Ecuatorial. *Informe de la Encuesta de Seroprevalencia del VIH en Guinea Ecuatorial, 2004.* Guinea Ecuatorial: 2004.
Sierra Leone	2005 survey. Sierra Leone: First post-war countrywide survey shows 1.5 percent HIV prevalence. IRIN, 2005. Available at: http://www.irinnews.org/report.aspx?reportid=57627 (accessed 8 September 2007).
South Africa	2005 survey. Shisana O, Rehle T, Simbayi LC, et al. *South African national HIV prevalence, HIV incidence, behaviour and communication survey. 2005.* Cape Town: HSRC Press, 2005. Available at: http://hsrcpress.ac.za/product.php?productid=2134 (accessed 8 September 2007).

Map of Africa

Annex Figure 1: Political map of Africa, 2007

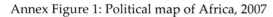

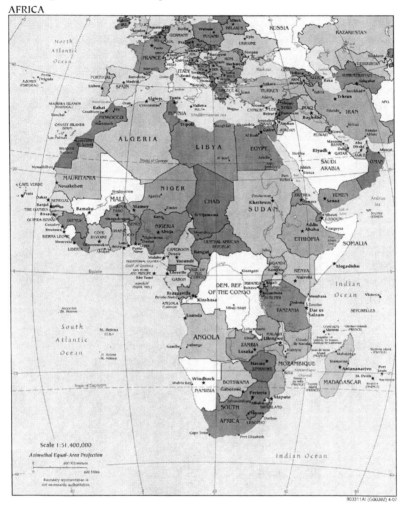

Source: Africa (political) 2007, University of Texas Libraries. Available at: http://www.lib.utexas.edu/maps/africa.html (accessed 24 September 2007).

215

Index

V

W

Y

Z